# COPING WITH Diabetes

# COPING WITH Diabetes

Sound, Compassionate Advice to Alleviate the Challenges of Type I and Type II Diabetes

ROBERT H. PHILLIPS, PH.D.

Avery
A MEMBER OF
PENGUIN PUTNAM INC.

Every effort has been made to ensure that the information contained in this book is complete and accurate. However, neither the publisher nor the author is engaged in rendering professional advice or services to the individual reader. The ideas, procedures, and suggestions contained in this book are not intended as a substitute for consulting with your physician. All matters regarding health require medical supervision. Neither the author nor the publisher shall be liable or responsible for any loss, injury, or damage allegedly arising from any information or suggestion in this book.

Most Avery books are available at special quantity discounts for bulk purchase for sales promotions, premiums, fund-raising, and educational needs. Special books or book excerpts also can be created to fit specific needs. For details, write Putnam Special Markets, 375 Hudson Street, New York, NY 10014.

Avery
a member of
Penguin Putnam Inc.
375 Hudson Street
New York, NY 10014
www.penguinputnam.com


Published simultaneously in Canada

Library of Congress Cataloging-in-Publication Data

Phillips, Robert H., date.
Coping with diabetes : Sound, Compassionate Advice to Alleviate
the Challenges of Type I and Type II Diabetes /
Robert H. Phillips.
p. cm.
Includes bibliographical references and index.
ISBN 0-89529-923-2
1. Diabetes—Popular works. I. Title.

RC660.4.P495 2000 00-32783
616.4'62—dc21

Printed in the United States of America
1 3 5 7 9 10 8 6 4 2

BOOK DESIGN BY JENNIFER ANN DADDIO

# Contents

## PART THREE
## Your Emotions



## PART FOUR
## Interacting with Other People

*This book is lovingly dedicated to my family—*

*my wife, Sharon, and my three sons,*

*Michael, Larry, and Steven;*

*my daughter-in-law Donna and her family;*

*my parents, sister, mother-in-law, nephews, niece, and favorite aunt;*

*and all my other relatives and in-laws—and to my friends.*

# Acknowledgments

Appreciative words of thanks must be accorded to some very special people who provided assistance in the preparation of this book. Thanks to Virginia Peragallo-Dittka for critical review, helpful suggestions, and belief in this project. Thanks to Peg Davis and the American Diabetes Association for being willing to provide insight and experience. Thanks to Paul Margulies, M.D., Howard Goldstein, M.D., and Richard Weiner, M.D., for their knowledgeable reviews of the manuscript and helpful suggestions. Thanks to Peggy Hahn for her superior editing and valuable comments. Thanks to Kathy Green for word processing and manuscript preparation. And finally, thanks for the support and efficiency introduced by Laura Shepherd of Penguin Putnam's Avery division.

# Foreword

I'm not happy with diabetes! I'd rather have just a hangnail or a mild headache or even a swollen ulna—but these were the cards dealt me when I was eight years old. Luckily, I am indentured to the work ethic, and that helps me cope in myriad ways.

This new book, *Coping with Diabetes*, by my longtime chum Robert Phillips, will also help. It's an information-packed volume that will be embraced by the 16 million people who suffer from this illness (and by their friends and family). Dr. Bob, a kind and erudite man of imperturbable placidity, has given us a marvelous guide to dealing with this chronic problem. He touches on every question you might have pertaining to diabetes.

So many friends of mine have suffered from this ailment—Dan Rowan, Jack Benny, Mel Torme, Ella Fitzgerald, Peggy Lee, Mary Tyler Moore, Ray Kroc (founder of McDonald's)—to name only a few. Fortunately, great strides are being made in finding a cure.

I was on the founding board for the Carousel Ball, a successful fund-raising charity that has given millions of dollars to the constant fight against the disease. Accolades and kudos go to Barbara and Marvin Davis for their phenomenal effort in helping children obtain their high hopes.

I've lived with diabetes for more than fifty years and I still play basketball twice a week. Exercise, diet, vitamins, insulin, a loving family, and a bright doctor all play a major role in this regard.

Again, my congratulations to Bob and his great new book. It's wonderful.

Gary Owens
Hollywood, California

*Gary Owens, a regular on NBC's* Rowan and Martin's Laugh-In *for all six of its award-winning seasons, has been a supervoice on more than three thousand animated cartoon episodes. He was inducted into the Radio Hall of Fame with Red Skelton, George Burns, and Garrison Keillor, and into the National Association of Broadcasters Hall of Fame with Carol Burnett, Ted Turner, and Larry King. His star is on the Hollywood Walk of Fame between those of Walt Disney and Betty White (6743 Hollywood Boulevard).*

# Introduction

The diagnosis of diabetes can have a major impact on you and your family. No kidding! Many people shudder when they just hear the word "diabetes." Fortunately, thanks to advances in modern medicine, diabetes can now be successfully managed, allowing individuals to lead long, productive, happy lives.

Certainly, there are many misconceptions, fears, concerns, and myths about diabetes and its treatment. Undoubtedly you have many questions about your condition. Some of them can be answered by physicians and other professionals. Others can be answered by books and articles on the subject. However, many questions cannot be answered. Why? Scientists just don't know all the answers.

In living with diabetes, you'll find yourself facing many important decisions. Initially, one of the most essential decisions you'll be making concerns how you can best become a partner in the treatment program that's going to help you, and how you can take control over the rest of your life, rather than letting life control you.

Heavy stuff? You bet it is! But that's why this book was written. Chock-full of information, suggestions, and strategies, this book will help you, your family, and your friends learn how to cope with diabetes.

The first two parts of the book present basic information about diabetes: what it is, what the symptoms are, what treatment techniques are available, and so on. The other parts of the book deal with important aspects of living with diabetes, including coping with emotions and living with others. We will explore each aspect in detail, and will examine many suggestions and strategies, as well as illustrative examples. In fact, a lot of the information you'll be reading can (and does!) apply to any chronic medical condition. In this book, however, the main focus is on your life with diabetes.

As you learn to cope with diabetes, it's important to realize that you're not alone; others are experiencing a lot of the same things that you're going through. This can be reassuring, but you should also remember that each person with diabetes experiences symptoms differently. Similarly, the psychological consequences of having diabetes vary from person to person. Your own life with diabetes—the way it affects you and the way you experience it—will not be exactly the same as anyone else's. You are a unique person. Therefore it will be up to *you* to use the suggestions and strategies presented in this book to help yourself cope as well as you possibly can. The goal of this book is to help you become an active person, rather than a passive patient.

Until such time as there is no longer a condition called diabetes, you'll have to live with it. I hope this book will help both you and your family do just that, and do it comfortably. Remember: You can *always* improve the quality of your life.

*Robert H. Phillips, Ph.D.*
*Center for Coping*
*Long Island, NY*

# PART ONE

# Diabetes—An Overview

## CHAPTER ONE

# What Is Diabetes?

Eddie, a forty-two-year-old salesman, had been feeling uncomfortable lately. He was always thirsty—it seemed like he could never get enough to drink—and he had to make endless trips to the bathroom, both during the day and at night. Plus, his vision was blurry, and he often had to rub his eyes to see clearly. Finally, Eddie decided to check in with his doctor, who gave him a complete physical examination and ordered a number of blood tests. After analyzing the results, the doctor gave Eddie the news: "You have diabetes." Eddie's concerned reaction was, "Oh, no! What am I going to do?"

An estimated 16 million Americans have diabetes, a chronic condition in which the body is unable to use energy from food efficiently. Nearly 800,000 more people are diagnosed with the disorder every year. Diabetes does not discriminate—it affects men and women of every age and race. As yet, there is no cure.

Anger, anxiety, and self-pity are common reactions to a diagnosis of diabetes. You may panic, or wonder if you'll be able to lead a "normal" life. Well, other people who are living with diabetes every day can tell you that you'll need to make some lifestyle changes. But these changes will help you control your symptoms and reduce the risk of long-term complications so you can lead a full, active life.

To understand the kind of impact diabetes will have on your life, you'll first have to understand what the disorder is and why it occurs. This chapter explains how the body normally processes food to produce energy, and how the three major types of diabetes affect the body's ability to use food for energy. It also outlines the symptoms of the disorder, and the long-term complications that can develop if you don't take measures to control your diabetes.

## How Does the Body Produce Energy?

Our bodies need energy to survive. Food provides us with that energy in the form of nutrients—carbohydrates, proteins, and fats. As food moves through the digestive system, from the mouth to the stomach to the intestines, it is broken down into these components. Carbohydrates are broken down in the small intestine into single sugar molecules called *simple sugars*. The most abundant of the simple sugars is *glucose*, which is the energy source for all of the body's cells. Glucose is absorbed through the intestinal walls into the bloodstream so it can circulate to the body's cells, tissues, and organs to nourish them. Once inside the body cells, glucose serves as a fuel to keep the body working efficiently. Any glucose that is not used immediately for energy is stored in the form of *glycogen*—long chains of sugar molecules—in the liver and muscle cells for future use.

Under normal circumstances, blood glucose levels are relatively stable. During periods before meals, blood sugar is comparatively low. After food is eaten, the concentration of glucose in the blood rises, as carbohydrates are digested and glucose is released into the bloodstream. But a healthy human body will always keep blood sugar levels from rising too high or falling too low.

# The Rise and Fall of Blood Sugar Levels

The pancreas is a small gland, weighing less than eight ounces, that secretes two hormones necessary for energy production. Hormones are chemical messengers that travel through the bloodstream and help regulate body activities. Within the pancreas are more than 100,000 clusters of cells called *islets of Langerhans,* first discovered by Paul Langerhans in 1869. About 75 percent of these cells are beta cells, which produce the hormone insulin. The other 25 percent, known as alpha cells, release the hormone glucagon. Together, these hormones regulate blood glucose. Insulin lowers blood sugar by allowing glucose to move from the blood into the cells, while glucagon stimulates the release of glucose into the blood.

The body is able to absorb glucose ten times faster with the help of insulin than without it. Not only does insulin enable the body's cells to use sugar (as well as other nutrients such as fats and proteins), but it also helps the body's tissues to store the nutrients that are circulating in the bloodstream after a meal. For example, insulin stimulates the enzyme *glycogen synthase,* which aids in manufacturing glycogen from glucose for storage. This removes excess glucose from the blood, keeping the level of sugar balanced. If insulin is low, the liver may not be able to store the excess sugar, and the glucose level in the bloodstream may continue to rise.

When you eat, your blood sugar level rises, and your pancreas immediately secretes insulin in order to keep the level from rising too high. Insulin helps body cells properly absorb and use glucose for energy by attaching to the outside of the cells on special sites called insulin receptors. The action is much like a key that is inserted into a lock—insulin unlocks the cell membrane and enables the glucose to enter. Once the glucose has entered the cell, it is metabolized, or "burned," by the cells for energy.

The concentration of glucose in the blood determines how much insulin or glucagon is released. As the concentration of sugar in the blood starts to rise, the beta cells in the pancreas begin to secrete more insulin. In response to insulin, the body cells take up more glucose from the blood, causing the blood glucose level to decrease. Liver cells also take up much of the glucose for storage as glycogen. When blood glucose returns to a normal range, the beta cells stop secreting insulin.

Between meals or during heavy exercise, the blood glucose level dips below a set point, and the alpha cells in the pancreas respond by secreting glucagon. Glucagon causes liver cells to break glycogen down into glucose, which is released into the bloodstream. Then, when the blood glucose level returns to the set point, the alpha cells lose their stimulus to produce glucagon.

## What Is Diabetes Mellitus?

Diabetes mellitus occurs when there is not enough insulin in the blood or when the body's cells do not respond properly to insulin. Remember that, without insulin, glucose cannot get into cells. This means that although glucose still circulates in the bloodstream, the body's cells can't absorb it and use it for fuel. As a result, they become starved for energy and begin to burn proteins and fats for fuel.

Because glucose is not absorbed by the body's cells, it remains in the bloodstream. As sugar continues to enter the bloodstream from dietary sources or from the liver's supply of glycogen, the concentration of sugar in the blood reaches abnormally high levels. Eventually, blood sugar levels rise so high that some of the excess sugar "spills" into the urine and passes out of the body. (Normally, glucose is not excreted through the urine.) High blood sugar levels resulting from uncontrolled diabetes can lead to serious complications.

### WHAT ARE THE SYMPTOMS OF DIABETES?

The symptoms of diabetes are not always apparent. In fact, some people who have diabetes may not even know it. For these people, the diagnosis is made during a routine physical or an evaluation for some other medical problem. However, for many other people, chronically high blood sugar levels cause noticeable symptoms that are characteristic of diabetes.

These symptoms may develop over a short period of time or they may appear gradually.

### *Frequent Urination (Polyuria)*

The kidneys are essential organs in the body's excretory system, which has the job of removing waste products from the blood and eliminating them from the body. When blood filters through the kidneys, water and valuable solutes—including glucose, salts, and amino acids (the building blocks of protein)—are reabsorbed into the bloodstream, while waste products are removed from the blood and excreted in the urine.

*Glycosuria,* or the presence of sugar in the urine, usually indicates that blood glucose levels are too high. In the person with diabetes, blood sugar levels rise so high that the kidneys are unable to reabsorb the excess glucose, which then spills into the urine. The fluids your body needs maintain proper fluid levels are pulled from the bloodstream along with the sugar, and are also eliminated by the kidneys into the urine. This results in large volumes of urine and more frequent urination.

### *Excessive Thirst (Polydipsia)*

Thirst depends on the body's blood volume and the concentration of substances in the blood. The frequent loss of large volumes of fluids causes blood volume to decrease, and the brain perceives this as a sign of dehydration. The natural response is thirst—fluid intake returns blood volume to a more normal level.

Drinking fluids that contain sugars (such as soda or orange juice) can exacerbate excessive thirst. As the digestive system continues to absorb glucose from dietary sources, the blood glucose concentration rises even higher, causing more frequent urination, which in turn causes excessive thirst . . . and the vicious cycle continues.

### *Frequent or Excessive Hunger (Polyphagia)*

The third symptom of the "poly" trio is polyphagia, which literally means "much hunger." As we discussed earlier, the person with diabetes is not able to use glucose from food as a source of energy. Because the body can't consume sufficient calories from dietary carbohydrates, the brain thinks the body is hungry. However, eating more food does not mean that more glucose will get into the cells. Instead, more food will cause blood sugar levels to rise higher.

### *Weight Loss*

You've already learned how high blood sugar can cause excessive hunger. But you may be surprised to learn that weight loss can accompany this symptom, even if the person with diabetes eats more than usual. This occurs because calories are lost as excessive sugar is eliminated in the urine. Unable to get energy from the blood sugar, the body turns to reserve fat supplies for energy. As the body burns fat—and the calories from fat—the person with diabetes loses weight. This type of weight loss is often symptomatic of type 1 diabetes.

### *Blurred Vision*

Early in the development of diabetes, before blood sugar is controlled, many people experience blurred vision. This happens because high blood sugar causes a buildup of fluid within the eye, which changes the shape of the eye's lens. After blood sugar is stabilized, the blurred vision resolves, although it may recur with another prolonged increase in blood sugar levels. Blurred vision is not a permanent change (you don't need eyeglasses at this point!). However, the problem should be corrected, because it can become more pronounced over the long-term.

### *Fatigue*

Fatigue is a very common symptom of diabetes. Remember that glucose is the body's main source of energy and that, without insulin, glucose can't enter the body's cells to be used as fuel. Instead, sugar remains in the bloodstream and some may be excreted in the urine. Clearly, the glucose is not going where it's needed, and the kidneys are essentially throwing away this important end product of digestion.

Fatigue can range from mild to severe. Mild fatigue is very often overlooked or attributed to other factors, such as overwork, stress, or age. However, extreme fatigue can interfere with a person's ability to perform normally his or her daily activities.

### *Confused Thinking*

High blood sugar can interfere with your ability to think clearly. You may feel a little disoriented about what you're doing. You may have more difficulty working or studying. You may experience more irritability and moodiness because of high blood sugar.

### *Recurring Infections*

People with chronic high blood glucose also run a greater risk of developing infections. High blood sugar levels decrease the effectiveness of the immune system, so it can't fight off many of the invading viruses, bacteria, and fungi that cause infections. Plus, bacteria and fungi thrive on sugar—they flourish in the body if the immune system can't destroy them first.

The most common infections that affect women with diabetes are vaginal yeast infections caused by an overgrowth of the yeast organism *Candida albicans.* Although yeast infections can be treated with prescription or over-the-counter creams and suppositories, they will recur unless blood sugar levels are properly controlled. Men may also develop yeast infections, usually in the groin area; however, yeast infections do not occur as frequently in men. Other infections that may be associated with high blood sugar include urinary tract infections, which are also more common in women than in men, infections in wounds, and infections in the gums or in the extremities, most commonly the feet.

Sometimes, infections develop as a result of other complications of diabetes. For example, poor circulation, a common complication of diabetes, increases the chances of infection and damage to extremities.

## Types of Diabetes

Diabetes is not one disease, but rather a general term for a group of disorders that results from the body's inefficiency in using glucose. The different types of diabetes are classified according to the underlying physical causes of the problem. In general, all individuals with diabetes have insulin problems.

The three main types of diabetes are: *type 1 diabetes,* in which the body produces an insufficient amount of insulin; *type 2 diabetes,* in which the body does not respond properly to the insulin that's produced; and *gestational diabetes,* which occurs only during pregnancy. In addition to the three major classifications of diabetes, medical conditions other than diabetes—as well as some medications—may cause *secondary diabetes,* which can result in a decreased production of insulin by the pancreas.

## TYPE 1 DIABETES

Type 1 diabetes was once known as *juvenile diabetes* because it's usually diagnosed in children and adolescents, although it can be diagnosed at any age. It has often been referred to as insulin-dependent diabetes; however, the trend seems to be moving toward simply calling the disorder type 1 diabetes.

In this type of diabetes, the beta cells of the pancreas produce very minimal amounts of insulin or no insulin at all. Since people with type 1 diabetes cannot produce insulin, they are unable to use glucose from food for fuel, and their cells become starved for energy. It is estimated that type 1 diabetes affects 10 to 15 percent of all people with diabetes.

When insulin is not available to help cells absorb glucose, the body has to burn fat as an alternate energy source. The breakdown of fat produces *ketones,* which begin to accumulate in the bloodstream and spill over into the urine as more and more fat is burned as fuel. High levels of ketones in the bloodstream cause the blood to become acidic, a dangerous condition known as *diabetic ketoacidosis* (DKA). The symptoms of DKA include excessive thirst, excessive urination, weight loss, nausea and vomiting, fatigue, and abdominal pain. Without medical intervention, DKA can progress to coma within several hours. Fortunately, careful monitoring of blood glucose levels and ketone levels in the urine can prevent DKA. The problem can also be corrected with insulin injections, especially if diagnosed early.

Because people with type 1 diabetes cannot produce insulin, they require daily insulin injections (often two or more a day) in order to survive. Insulin is not effective in pill form because stomach acid will destroy the insulin before it can do its work. People with type 1 diabetes must also monitor their blood glucose closely to make sure they're controlling their blood sugar levels effectively.

### *What Causes Type 1 Diabetes?*

Although the cause of type 1 diabetes is still unclear, it's believed that the condition is caused by an autoimmune disorder. In other words, the immune system perceives the body's own tissues to be the "enemy," and therefore attacks and destroys healthy cells. In this type of diabetes, *autoantibodies* produced by the immune system attack the insulin-producing beta cells in the pancreas. This causes insulin production to decrease dramatically, and in many cases to cease altogether.

Some experts believe that viruses may cause type 1 diabetes. Viral infections such as mumps, German measles, and Coxsackie viruses might trigger the development of the antibodies that cause type 1 diabetes.

## TYPE 2 DIABETES

Type 2 diabetes affects some 85 to 90 percent of all people with diabetes. This type of diabetes is generally—but not always—diagnosed in adults over forty years of age. It is most often diagnosed in people who are obese; approximately 85 percent of people diagnosed with type 2 diabetes are overweight at the time of diagnosis.

Type 2 diabetes has also been referred to as *non-insulin-dependent diabetes* because people who have the condition can still produce some insulin. However, individuals with type 2 diabetes may not produce enough insulin, or their cells are resistant to the amount of insulin that is produced. In either case, the body's ability to use glucose for energy is reduced. Because the person with type 2 diabetes can still produce some insulin, this type of diabetes does not result in diabetic ketoacidosis.

Type 2 diabetes usually develops gradually over a period of years, and the symptoms are not as noticeable as in type 1 diabetes. Often, the diagnosis of type 2 diabetes is made during a routine physical examination. Because the symptoms (if there are any) may go unnoticed, it's practically impossible to pinpoint exactly when an individual developed the disorder.

In many cases, type 2 diabetes can be managed through a lifelong program of diet, exercise, and weight control. However, the disorder may progress so that oral medication or insulin injections are necessary to bring blood sugar levels under control. Oral medications may be helpful in stimulating the pancreas to secrete more insulin or to improve the way in which the body uses insulin. Type 2 individuals who take insulin are referred to as "insulin-requiring" individuals.

### *What Causes Type 2 Diabetes?*

Like type 1 diabetes, type 2 diabetes does not have one certain cause. Usually, the disorder results from a combination of factors. The key to pinpointing the cause to type 2 diabetes lies in understanding why insulin produced by the pancreas is not properly used.

A primary factor in the development of type 2 diabetes appears to be genetics. The role that heredity plays in type 2 diabetes is much more apparent than it is in type 1 diabetes. Obesity is another contributing factor in the development of type 2 diabetes. It's estimated that 80 to 90 percent of people with type 2 diabetes are obese. Many consume high-fat diets with a high concentration of refined foods, and they tend to lead sedentary lifestyles. As the body accumulates excess fat, the cells become increasingly resistant to the effects of insulin. Consequently, the pancreas must secrete more and more insulin in order to remove glucose from the bloodstream. As insulin resistance progresses, blood insulin levels become chronically elevated, and this condition can lead to diabetes.

## GESTATIONAL DIABETES

Changes in levels and types of hormones produced during pregnancy can cause insulin resistance, increasing the body's requirements for insulin. This may cause previously healthy women to develop *gestational diabetes* during pregnancy. Gestational diabetes affects 3 to 4 percent of pregnant women. It is usually detected by a blood glucose test given after the twenty-fourth week of pregnancy.

It is important to identify and to treat gestational diabetes effectively, because left untreated the condition increases the risk of birth defects, high birth weight, and complications during delivery. If there is too much glucose in the mother's blood during the last half of the pregnancy, the baby may grow too large to be delivered safely. This is called macrosomia, and may increase the need for delivery by cesarean section. Infants born to mothers with gestational diabetes also have a greater chance of developing weight problems later in life. Also, women with gestational diabetes may develop other health problems, such as pregnancy-induced hypertension (high blood pressure). If left untreated, PIH can develop into preeclampsia, which is characterized by high blood pressure, protein in the urine, sudden weight gain, and swelling of the face and hands. Women with gestational diabetes need to be closely monitored by a health professional to avoid these dangerous complications.

In most cases, women with gestational diabetes have no previous history of either type 1 or type 2 diabetes. The condition usually goes away after the baby is born. However, a woman who has gestational diabetes during pregnancy has an increased risk of developing type 2 diabetes later in life.

### *What Causes Gestational Diabetes?*

Gestational diabetes is related to insulin resistance, rather than insufficient insulin. Women with this condition actually have plenty of insulin in their blood. The problem is that insulin's action is partially blocked by hormones secreted by the placenta. These hormones, including estrogen, cortisol, and human placental lactogen (HPL), are essential to a healthy pregnancy. However, they interfere with the insulin that is released by the pancreas. As a woman's pregnancy progresses, the placenta increases in size to nourish the developing fetus, and more hormones are produced, increasing the degree of insulin resistance. When insulin from the pancreas can't overcome the effects of placental hormones, gestational diabetes results.

## SECONDARY DIABETES

In some instances, diabetes results from medical conditions or medications that damage the pancreas or interfere with its production of insulin. For example, chronic or severe pancreatitis, a condition in which the pancreas is inflamed, can damage the ability of the pancreas to produce insulin. Pancreatic tumors can also damage the pancreas, resulting in decreased insulin production.

Certain endocrine diseases may produce an excess of hormones that block the action of insulin produced by the pancreas. And drugs such as prednisone, a powerful anti-inflammatory used for severe arthritis, lupus, and other conditions, can suppress insulin secretion or inhibit insulin's actions.

Fortunately, diabetes caused by medications or other medical problems can often be reversed when the individual stops taking the medications or when the medical problems are resolved. However, some experts speculate that an underlying predisposition to diabetes must have existed in the first place for the diabetes to have developed.

## What Are the Long-Term Complications of Diabetes?

Prolonged periods of high blood sugar increase the risk of complications in people with diabetes. For example, a high concentration of glucose in the blood can damage blood vessels and nerves throughout the body, which can cause various disorders, including:

- Eye problems, such as *diabetic retinopathy,* which results from damage to the small blood vessels that supply blood and oxygen to the eyes; *glaucoma,* in which pressure inside the eyes increases and damages the optic nerves; and *cataracts,* which are opaque particles inside the lens of the eyes that cloud vision.
- Kidney disease, or *diabetic nephropathy,* caused by damage to the small blood vessels that are vital to the kidneys' ability to filter blood.
- Nerve disorders, known as *diabetic neuropathies,* which can damage the insulation surrounding the nerves, reducing the speed at which nerves travel throughout the body.

- Cardiovascular problems, including *hypertension* (high blood pressure); hardening of the arteries, also called *atherosclerosis*; heart attack; and stroke.
- Foot and lower leg problems, or *peripheral vascular disease*, caused by poor circulation.

Most of the conditions listed above result from years of chronic high blood sugar levels. This is why it's so important to take good care of yourself by keeping your blood sugar levels controlled and getting regular checkups to catch the earliest signs of complications before they become real problems. You'll learn in chapter 11 more about common problems associated with diabetes.

## Who Gets Diabetes?

Although diabetes can affect anyone of any age, sex, or race, it's clear that certain people are more prone to developing the disease than are others. While nobody can predict who will get diabetes, some definite risk factors have been identified. For example, heredity has been shown to play a major role in the development of type 2 diabetes. In fact, 35 to 40 percent of siblings and one third of children of people with type 2 diabetes will develop the disorder or associated problems with glucose metabolism at some point in their lives. By comparison, people with type 1 diabetes are less likely to have family members also affected by the disorder.

Obesity and sedentary lifestyle, which often go hand in hand, are also strong risk factors for type 2 diabetes. As you've already learned, too much extra weight can cause the body cells to become resistant to the effects of insulin. And age appears to play a part in the development of type 2 diabetes, since this type of diabetes affects one in five individuals over the age of sixty-five. This seems to occur, in part, because many people gain weight as they grow older.

Women who have a history of gestational diabetes or who have given birth to babies weighing more than nine pounds are also susceptible to developing type 2 diabetes. Gestational diabetes is diagnosed in approximately 135,000 women each year. Of these women, it's estimated that 40 percent will develop type 2 diabetes within fifteen years after the occurrence of gestational diabetes.

## What Is the Prognosis for Diabetes?

The prognosis for living with diabetes is excellent. Ongoing research and improved technology and treatment techniques are significantly reducing the incidence of serious complications—and improved medical care means improved quality of life for people who are affected by diabetes. While doctors can't predict the course that the disease will take in any particular individual, they will certainly agree that treatment makes a big difference, so the earlier you begin treatment for your diabetes, the more you can improve your prognosis.

Your commitment to taking good care of yourself is the most valuable indicator of how well you will be able to control your diabetes. When you make an effort to know all there is to know about your diabetes, you will be more likely to take an active part in managing the condition. Patient participation in treatment is more important in diabetes than in almost any other disease. Recognizing that you *do* have an impact on how diabetes affects your body and your lifestyle, and taking the appropriate steps to control your diabetes, will minimize the risk that you'll develop serious long-term complications—and that will allow you to lead a long and healthy life.

# CHAPTER TWO

# How Is Diabetes Diagnosed?

As you learned in the last chapter, diabetes may or may not be accompanied by obvious symptoms. In some cases, any number of symptoms become apparent very rapidly and are impossible to ignore. For example, when a patient complains of frequent urination, excessive thirst, and sudden weight loss, the physician should immediately suspect diabetes. But this is not always the case. Some people who have diabetes don't even suspect they have it, because they haven't experienced any overt symptoms. In such cases, diabetes is discovered quite by accident during a routine examination.

The only sure way to determine that you have diabetes is to have your doctor measure your blood sugar levels. This can be done through one of several different blood tests. Some tests require you to fast, and are usually done in the morning; some can be given at any time of the day, even if you've eaten. If your blood sugar levels are too high, it's possible that diabetes is the cause. However, your doctor may have you repeat a blood glucose test or take a different test to confirm a definite diagnosis.

You may be wondering why so many tests exist to diagnose the same disease, or how high your blood sugar level has to be for your doctor to make a diagnosis. This chapter will help clear up some of the mystery that surrounds diabetes testing by explaining what's involved in each of the different diagnostic tests, including what you should and shouldn't do before your test.

## Who Should Be Tested for Diabetes?

Testing for diabetes is certainly a lifesaver when symptoms of the disorder have become obvious. However, individuals who are at high risk should not wait until they experience symptoms to be tested for diabetes. Screening tests can be performed on people who do not have symptoms of diabetes. They are inexpensive, and many require as little as a drop of blood from your fingertip. All people over forty-five years of age should be screened for diabetes—even if they do not have symptoms of the disease—and screening should be repeated every three years thereafter. Individuals under the age of forty-five should be screened for diabetes if they have one or more of the following risk factors for diabetes:

- Obesity
- High-risk ethnic background, including: African American, Hispanic, and Native American groups
- A parent or sibling who has diabetes
- History of gestational diabetes or delivery of a baby weighing over nine pounds
- Hypertension
- History of impaired glucose tolerance

In addition, all pregnant women should be screened for gestational diabetes between the twenty-fourth and twenty-eighth weeks of pregnancy.

# How Are Blood Glucose Levels Measured?

The amount of sugar concentrated in the blood is measured in units called milligrams per deciliter (mg/dl), or milligrams of glucose per 100 milliliters of blood. The normal "fasting" level of sugar in the blood—usually before breakfast or after another length of time when no calories are taken in by eating—ranges from 60 to 115 mg/dl in a person who does not have diabetes. After eating, the concentration of blood sugar increases, although it usually does not rise above 180 mg/dl in a healthy person. Over a period of two to four hours, blood sugar returns to the body's normal baseline. There is no such thing as a constant blood sugar level; it is normal for the concentration of glucose in the blood to vary. However, the variations that occur in people without diabetes are not as marked as the variations in people with diabetes.

# Blood Tests to Diagnose Diabetes

Diagnostic tests are used to confirm a diagnosis of diabetes if there are symptoms or other indicators of the disease. For diagnostic tests, the doctor draws one or more samples of blood and sends them to a lab for analysis. Diagnostic tests vary according to cost, accuracy, and ease of administration.

There are a number of different types of blood tests that can be used to diagnose diabetes. These include the *fasting plasma glucose (FPG) test,* which is given after the patient has fasted for at least eight hours; the *random plasma glucose test,* for which the patient does not have to fast; and the *oral glucose tolerance test* (OGTT), which also requires fasting and is administered after the patient has ingested a special glucose-containing solution. In addition, a doctor will use the *glucose challenge test* to determine if a woman has gestational diabetes. And professionals are still debating the value of the *glycosylated hemoglobin* ($HbA1_c$) *test* in diagnosing diabetes (see the inset on page 24).

You may be wondering why doctors use blood tests rather than urine tests to diagnose diabetes, since one of the warning signs of diabetes is the presence of glucose in the urine. While high urine glucose levels alert doctors to the possibility of diabetes, urine tests are just not as accurate as blood tests. This is because the level of blood sugar that causes glucose to spill into the urine is different for each person. Even though a person's blood sugar levels are high, glucose may not appear in the urine, or it may be present in minute amounts. So urine tests are useful in detecting the presence of diabetes, but blood glucose tests are necessary to make a definite diagnosis.

Let's take a closer look at what's involved in diagnostic testing for diabetes.

## FASTING PLASMA GLUCOSE (FPG) TEST

The fasting plasma glucose test is given after the patient has fasted for at least eight hours, usually overnight. "Fasting" means not taking in any foods or drinks that contain calories. Then a blood sample is taken in a laboratory or in the doctor's office to measure blood glucose levels.

Normally, adults who do not have diabetes have a fasting blood sugar level that's less than 110 mg/dl. Fasting levels ranging from 110 to 126 mg/dl are considered abnormal, but are not high enough for a diagnosis of diabetes. Blood sugar levels in this range indicate *impaired glucose tolerance* (IGT), previously called borderline, chemical, or latent diabetes. An individual with IGT is considered to be at increased risk of developing type 2 diabetes in the future. Management includes a program of healthy eating and exercise, in combination with frequent screenings for diabetes, which can help prevent IGT from developing into type 2 diabetes.

An FPG measurement greater than 126 mg/dl indicates diabetes. To make a definite diagnosis, doctors usually require a second fasting plasma glucose test—given on a different day—that measures over 126 mg/dl.

## RANDOM PLASMA GLUCOSE TEST

The random plasma glucose test, also called the *casual plasma glucose test,* measures blood glucose levels at any given time. This is the simplest test for diabetes because it can be administered whether or not the person has had anything to eat or drink. If the person being tested has random plasma glucose results of 200 mg/dl or higher and also exhibits symptoms of diabetes (excessive hunger and thirst, frequent urination, weight loss, and so on), then diabetes may be diagnosed. The diagnosis can be confirmed through repeat testing on a different day.

## ORAL GLUCOSE TOLERANCE TEST (OGTT)

The oral glucose tolerance test is more complicated than either the fasting plasma glucose or random plasma glucose tests, so it is not routinely used to diagnose diabetes. Usually, doctors rely on the OGTT when other tests have not conclusively indicated diabetes, or if it's believed that gestational diabetes is causing higher-than-normal blood sugar levels.

For reliable OGTT results, the person being tested must not have any other illness—not even a cold! A fast of at least ten hours (but no more than sixteen hours) is necessary before the test. A person taking the OGTT should not drink coffee or smoke on the day the test is administered.

The OGTT measures blood glucose levels five times over a period of three hours. First, an initial blood sugar is drawn to measure fasting plasma glucose levels, and then the person being tested is given 75 grams of glucose (or 100 grams for pregnant women) in a sweet-tasting solution. Blood sugar levels are measured at thirty minutes and at one, two, and three hours after the solution is given. In a person who does not have diabetes, blood sugar levels rise after drinking the glucose solution but fall quickly back to normal as insulin enables body cells to absorb glucose from the bloodstream. In a person with diabetes, on the other hand, glucose levels rise higher than normal and take a much longer time to decrease.

A person whose two-hour glucose level is less than or equal to 100 mg/dl is said to have a normal response. When the two-hour glucose level is greater than or equal to 140 mg/dl but less than 200 mg/dl, the person is said to have impaired glucose tolerance (see page 22). A diagnosis of diabetes is made when the OGTT results show that the blood glucose level at two hours is equal to or more than 200 mg/dl and is confirmed by a second test on another day.

### GLUCOSE TOLERANCE TEST

The glucose tolerance test is used to diagnose gestational diabetes in women who are pregnant. It is given between the twenty-fourth and twenty-eighth weeks of pregnancy. The woman being tested is given a glucose solution to drink, and her blood glucose level is measured one hour later. A level above 200 mg/dl usually indicates diabetes. An oral glucose tolerance test is usually required to make a definite diagnosis.

---

## What Is $HbA1_c$ Testing?

The glycosylated hemoglobin test ($HbA1_c$) test is a relatively new method for tracking blood glucose levels that also offers the potential for diagnosing diabetes. This test measures levels of glycosylated hemoglobin, also known as hemoglobin $A1_c$. Hemoglobin is a protein-iron compound in red blood cells that enables them to carry oxygen from the lungs to all of the body's tissues. Glycosylated hemoglobin forms when sugar becomes attached to hemoglobin molecules. The more glucose in the blood, the more hemoglobin becomes glycosylated. Hemoglobin molecules remain glycosylated until the red blood cell dies, usually after about three months.

Experts who advocate using the $HbA1_c$ test to diagnose diabetes argue that it is more convenient than standard blood tests for diabetes because it can be administered at any time, whether or not the person being tested has eaten. Those who are opposed to using the test for diagnosis point out that it's more expensive than other blood tests, and it is also more difficult to perform accurately.

In addition, although elevated $HbA1_c$ indicates impaired glucose tolerance (IGT) or diabetes, people with IGT or diabetes *can* have normal $HbA1_c$ levels. As such, the absence of $HbA1_c$ does not always mean an absence of diabetes.

Regardless of its controversial benefit as a diagnostic tool, the glycosylated hemoglobin test has been proven effective for tracking blood sugar levels over several weeks. This is very useful for defining overall patterns in blood glucose control. To learn more about the value of the HbA1c test as a glucose monitoring tool, see chapter 5.

---

## Type 1 or Type 2?

A diagnosis of diabetes is, of course, the first important step toward ensuring that the patient will receive proper medical care. More important still is a correct diagnosis of the type of diabetes, because the doctor needs to develop an appropriate treatment program based on whether the person is insulin deficient or insulin resistant. As you have already learned, a person with type 1 diabetes will need insulin right away, whereas a person with type 2 diabetes may be able to maintain lower blood glucose levels with a healthy diet, a program of regular exercise, and possibly oral diabetes medication.

In making a diagnosis of either type 1 or type 2 diabetes, the doctor will take into account factors such as age, weight, heredity, the presence of symptoms, and the presence of ketones in the urine. Generally speaking, people with type 1 diabetes are younger than thirty years old and are relatively thin. These people typically have had diabetic ketoacidosis or high levels of ketones in their urine. On the other hand, individuals with type 2 diabetes are usually older than thirty years of age, and at least 90 percent of the time they are overweight.

Unfortunately, misdiagnosis can—and does—occur. For example, what if the person with diabetes is over forty years old and slender? Or sixteen years old and overweight? In cases such as these, a variety of lab tests can provide the information necessary to make a definite diagnosis of the particular type of diabetes. For example, when a urine or blood test shows large amounts of ketones, then the person definitely has type 1 diabetes. Also, because type 1 diabetes is known to be an autoimmune disease, the person can be tested to see if he or she has the autoantibodies that are characteristic of this condition. By the same token, type 2 diabetes is more likely to be diagnosed in people with high triglycerides and low HDL cholesterol levels, which are typical in cases of insulin resistance. A high level of uric acid also indicates type 2 diabetes.

## Summing It All Up

Diabetes is not always accompanied by obvious symptoms. That's why screening for diabetes can be so important for people who are at high risk of developing the condition. Individuals who have one or more risk factors for diabetes—including obesity, a high-risk background, or a family history of diabetes—should not wait until they experience symptoms to be tested for diabetes.

Blood tests are the only sure way to diagnose diabetes. A doctor may use either the fasting plasma glucose test, the random plasma glucose test, or the oral glucose tolerance test to determine if diabetes is present. If blood sugar levels are too high, there is a strong probability that diabetes is the cause.

Now that you know how diabetes is diagnosed, let's take a look at treatment for the condition. Turn the page to learn about the basics of diabetes management.

## CHAPTER THREE

# How Is Diabetes Treated?

Now that you've learned a little about how diabetes is diagnosed, the more important question is "What can be done to treat it?" Some people worry that once you have diabetes, you can't do much to stop it from progressing into a more severe disease. This couldn't be further from the truth. In most cases, a comprehensive treatment program can help you to live a comfortable and satisfying life.

Treatment for diabetes varies from person to person and depends on the type of diabetes. This chapter will discuss the factors that all diabetes treatment programs have in common, and the goals that people with diabetes should aim for when they undertake treatment. You will also learn about the support network of medical professionals—known as the treatment team—that design and implement the diabetes treatment program.

## Goals of Treatment

Because abnormally high blood sugar levels are characteristic of all types of diabetes, the main goal of any treatment program is to bring glucose levels down to as close to normal as possible (the American Diabetes Association recommends 80 to 120 mg/dl before meals). By keeping your blood sugar level within a normal range, you can prevent short-term complications of diabetes, such as hypoglycemia (low blood sugar) and hyperglycemia (high blood sugar), and greatly reduce your risk of developing long-term complications, including kidney disease, cardiovascular disease, and nerve damage. Following the guidelines listed below will help you achieve and maintain your target glucose level.

- Take any insulin or diabetes medication exactly as prescribed by your physician.
- Maintain a normal body weight. If you are overweight, lose weight. Being overweight places additional stress on all parts of the body and adds to the pressure for insulin production. In addition to contributing to metabolic control, weight loss will decrease your risk of cardiovascular disease and hypertension.
- Follow a regular program of exercise. Exercise provides a foundation for good metabolic control and helps control weight and stress. It also has significant benefits for cardiorespiratory fitness.
- Take proper care of your eyes, teeth, skin, and feet. This is important because any infection, especially in these areas, can disrupt diabetes control.
- Don't smoke. Smoking usually increases the risk of vascular disorders and heart disease—risks already heightened in diabetes. Smoking has a negative effect on arteries, small blood vessels, blood pressure, and circulation, thus contributing to atherosclerosis, hypertension, and coronary artery disease.

## Your Treatment Team

Diabetes treatment can be a complicated affair. Because each individual is unique, there is no single treatment program that's appropriate for everyone. Achieving lower blood sugar levels may require a combination of insulin and/or oral diabetes medications, a comprehensive weight loss program, an appropriate exercise regimen, and a balanced eating plan that's designed to meet your specific nutritional needs. In addition, should you develop any of the complications associated with diabetes, you will need medical treatment for that particular problem. But your doctor alone cannot be an expert in every area. Diabetes care requires a group of skilled professionals with different areas of expertise. Together, these health-care professionals are known as your treatment team.

The focus of this kind of integrated care is on you, the patient, and the aim of the group is to help you follow the guidelines outlined on page 28. Emphasis is given to education and counseling, rather than medical treatment alone, so you can learn to manage your diabetes when you're away from the doctor's office.

Let's take a few moments to discuss the members of your treatment team.

## PHYSICIAN

Your primary-care physician takes responsibility for your overall health. Oftentimes, he or she is your family physician or internist. In some cases, your primary-care physician may be a diabetologist or endocrinologist—a doctor who has special training in caring for people with diabetes. Whether or not your doctor is a diabetes specialist, he or she will be in charge of your care on a regular basis.

Your primary-care physician will determine what is the best blood sugar range for you, and will prescribe any medications that you may need to bring your blood glucose level under control. During your regular appointments, expect the doctor to give you a physical examination, take a medical history, run laboratory tests, and fine-tune your treatment program.

If you develop any of the complications of diabetes, your primary-care physician will refer you to a specialist who can oversee treatment of the complication. For skin problems, you will be referred to a dermatologist; for nerve problems, a neurologist; for digestive problems, a gastroenterologist or neurologist; for foot problems, a podiatrist; and for eye problems, an ophthalmologist.

## DIABETES EDUCATOR

Diabetes educators are health professionals—including nurse practitioners, patient educators, and dietitians—who can teach you the important skills you need to effectively manage your diabetes. By getting to know you as an individual—assessing your school or work schedule, your day-to-day activities, and your eating habits—your diabetes educator can help you fit diabetes self-management into your everyday life.

Your diabetes educator will speak with you about controlling your blood sugar with proper nutrition and exercise, how insulin and oral diabetes medications work, how to test your blood sugar level, how to give yourself insulin shots if necessary, and when to take oral medications if they are prescribed for you. Because physical and emotional stress can have a big impact on your blood glucose levels, your diabetes educator may also teach you some effective strategies for managing stress in your life, such as meditation and imaging. (You'll find more information about stress management in chapter 24.)

## DIETITIAN

A registered dietitian (RD) is educated to understand nutrition, food science, and diet planning, and to deliver counsel and care to people with varying nutritional needs. Your RD will assess your nutritional status and work with you to develop and implement your individualized care plan. To ensure success, the dietitian will take into account your lifestyle and motivation to help you set realistic nutritional goals, and will also provide ongoing support so you'll stick with your program to achieve those goals.

## MENTAL HEALTH PROFESSIONAL

There's no doubt that learning to live with diabetes is a difficult adjustment. It's natural to feel sad, angry, or anxious, or to resist starting a lifelong treatment program. Many people find it necessary to reach out to someone who can help sort out all of the feelings that come along with a diagnosis of diabetes. This person may be a psychologist, psychiatrist, social worker, or counselor who has special training in helping people who are experiencing crises or difficult changes in their lives.

A mental-health professional can help you adjust to the lifestyle changes that occur after diagnosis by providing assistance in setting treatment goals and by supporting your efforts to manage your diabetes day by day.

## EXERCISE SPECIALIST

While exercise is recommended for everyone, the potential benefits for people with diabetes are so great that regular exercise is a *must* as part of any treatment program. Your exercise specialist will work in conjunction with other members of your treatment team to develop an appropriate exercise regimen for you. When designing your individualized program, your exercise specialist will take into account your age, weight, physical condition, level of fitness, and long-term goals, such as good control of blood sugar levels, weight loss, or cardiorespiratory fitness. Then the specialist will track your progress and evaluate—and possibly fine-tune—your exercise program.

## PHARMACIST

Your pharmacist provides you with your prescribed medication, and can also be very helpful in offering information and advice about insulin and other medications, as well as a wide variety of diabetes products—such as blood glucose monitors or insulin pumps—that may be part of your treatment program. It's important to develop a good relationship with your pharmacist. Make sure that he or she takes an interest in your medical needs, and is available to answer any questions you might have about your medications.

## Your Role in Treatment

Above all, *you* are the most important member of your treatment team because *you* are the one who lives with diabetes every day. It's up to you to monitor your blood glucose levels and to take any medications necessary to keep these levels within a normal range. And it's your job to make healthy food choices and to follow your exercise program. Ultimately, you are the person responsible for making important decisions about your care. Regardless of how many professionals are on your side, if you don't take steps to effectively manage your diabetes, you will be putting yourself at a greater risk of developing complications.

Keep in mind the importance of maintaining open, honest communication with all members of your treatment team. It's your responsibility to make these professionals aware of your questions and concerns. If you don't understand what you are told, or if you feel you are being given too much information at once, speak up! If you have doubts about a recommendation, or if you would like to learn about alternative treatment plans, let the appropriate person know. The members of your treatment team are there for you—they want you to live a comfortable and complication-free life.

## Developing an Individualized Treatment Program

You are a unique individual. To be effective, your diabetes treatment program must be designed specifically to meet your special needs. This means that you have to be involved in developing your care plan. By being an active participant in your treatment planning, you'll be able to tailor your program to fit your lifestyle.

In designing your treatment program, you and your health-care team will take into account numerous factors, including:

- The type of diabetes you have.
- The symptoms of diabetes, if any, that are apparent.
- Your age.
- Your weight.
- Your family and social situation.
- Your overall general health.
- How active you are.
- Your school or work schedule.
- What and when you like to eat.
- Other medical conditions you may have.
- Any complications that have developed.

Obviously, the type of diabetes you have is the most important factor in developing your diabetes care program. People with type 1 diabetes need multiple daily injections of insulin to survive, and they must monitor their blood glucose levels several times each day. Individuals who have type 2 diabetes, on the other hand, do not necessarily need insulin injections or other medications to control their blood sugar levels. Usually, one of the first goals of a treatment plan for type 2 diabetes is weight loss. In some cases, eating right and adopting an appropriate exercise plan is enough to manage this type of diabetes. For women with gestational diabetes, the first course of action is to implement a healthy diet plan in order to regulate blood sugar levels. If blood sugar cannot be controlled by diet alone, treatment with insulin may be necessary.

The end result of all this planning will be a complete treatment program that will enable you to keep good control over your blood glucose levels and prevent or minimize diabetes-related complications. Your complete diabetes care plan should include a list of short- and long-term goals, a list of medications (if you need them) that will help you keep your blood sugar levels controlled, a meal plan developed by your dietitian or nutritionist, guidelines for following an appropriate exercise regimen, and instructions on when you should visit your primary-care physician and other doctors.

# Components of Treatment Programs

Although managing your diabetes may seem like a momentous task at first, it's guaranteed to be well worth the effort. What you do today in terms of managing the disorder will affect your health and well-being in the future.

Regardless of the type of diabetes you have, you'll have to monitor your blood sugar daily, and keep your glucose levels controlled by eating right and exercising. If you have type 1 diabetes, you will definitely need insulin shots, so it's important that you understand how to give yourself injections, and that you are careful to take the proper doses at the same times each day. If you have type 2 diabetes, you may need to take insulin shots or oral diabetes medications if a good diet and exercise program is not adequate to keep your blood sugar levels under control.

Whatever treatment program is planned for your diabetes, the overall goal is the same. You want to control your blood sugar levels as much as possible to prevent or minimize both short-term and long-term complications. There are four components involved in all proper diabetes management programs: monitoring your blood glucose levels, following a healthy diet, implementing and following an exercise program, and knowing how and when to take any medications that your doctor prescribes.

## MONITORING YOUR BLOOD GLUCOSE LEVELS

Closely monitoring your blood glucose levels is one of the most important things you can do to keep your diabetes under control. By measuring your blood sugar levels each day, or several times each day, you'll be able to evaluate the efficacy of your diabetes treatment program. While a single slightly high or low measurement probably doesn't indicate a serious problem, several abnormal readings may be cause for concern. If your blood sugar level is consistently above or below your target measurement, then you'll most likely need to work with your health-care team to adjust one or more factors involved in your treatment program.

Blood glucose monitors are available for home use, so you don't have to make a trip to the doctor's office to get your blood sugar checked. You can purchase a monitor at most pharmacies with or without a prescription from your doctor. With recent advances in technology, many monitoring systems are now smaller, more reliable, and less expensive. Some devices can even store blood sugar readings for a few days or weeks. Ask your diabetes educator to help you choose a meter that is appropriate for your lifestyle.

In addition to a blood glucose monitor, you'll want to invest in a diabetes diary or notebook in which you can keep a record of your test results. Look for a diary that has spaces for you to jot down factors that may have affected your blood sugar levels, such as an illness or strenuous physical activity. Keeping track of your blood glucose levels in a diabetes diary will enable you to identify patterns that indicate a need to adjust your treatment program. A word of caution is in order here: If you should recognize a problem in your treatment program, consult your doctor before making any changes. *Never* try to modify your diabetes care plan without the guidance of a health-care professional.

How often you check your blood sugar levels depends on the type of diabetes you have, whether you are taking any medication for your diabetes, and how motivated you are to control your diabetes. Your doctor can help you establish a monitoring schedule that you'll be comfortable following.

You'll learn more about incorporating blood glucose monitoring into your diabetes care plan in chapter 5.

## MEAL PLANNING

Good nutrition is at the very foundation of treatment for all types of diabetes. Obviously, the most important aim of meal planning is to help you maintain blood glucose levels as close to normal as possible. But a sound diet will also help you achieve other goals such as weight loss and/or weight control, healthy blood cholesterol and triglyceride levels, and prevention of short-term and long-term complications of diabetes.

One of the key aspects involved in diabetes meal planning is the development of a diet that's low in fat and cholesterol. Too many high-fat foods will cause you to gain weight and will send your blood glucose and cholesterol levels soaring. Weight loss is a common goal for a great percentage of people with diabetes. Gradual weight loss will produce significant improvements in your blood glucose levels, which will greatly reduce your risk of developing cardiovascular disease. However, always remember the importance of balance in your diet. If your aim is to lose weight, you shouldn't restrict your diet too much, because too little food will cause your blood glucose levels to drop dramatically. This can cause hypoglycemia, which is a potentially dangerous short-term complication of diabetes. Your dietitian or nutritionist will be able to tell you how many calories you need each day to meet your energy needs, and will guide you in making nutritious food choices that will enable you to maximize your health.

If you take insulin injections or oral diabetes medication, it's very important that you time your meals appropriately. Insulin and other medications are designed to lower blood glucose, so if you don't eat soon enough after taking your medication, your blood sugar levels may drop too low, resulting in hypoglycemia.

You'll learn more about meal planning for diabetes in chapter 8.

## EXERCISE

If you don't already exercise regularly, now's the time to start! Exercise is good for everyone. It helps us look good and feel better about ourselves, and it increases cardiorespiratory fitness, aids in weight control, and improves muscle tone. For people with diabetes, exercise offers even greater benefits. Most important, regular exercise can help improve blood glucose control. Daily physical activity reduces the body's resistance to insulin and increases the body cells' sensitivity to insulin. Therefore, people with type 1 diabetes can keep tight control over their blood sugar levels with smaller amounts of insulin. The same goes for individuals with type 2 diabetes who need to take insulin or oral diabetes medications.

Another benefit of exercise is that it can help reduce blood fat levels, decreasing the risk of heart attack or stroke. Again, this is particularly crucial for people with diabetes, who are at greater risk of developing cardiovascular disease. Plus, a regular exercise program, in combination with your individualized diet plan, contributes to effective weight loss, which is especially important for many people with type 2 diabetes.

Before you begin any exercise program, you should schedule a complete physical to make sure that exercising is safe for you. Your physician or exercise specialist will help you develop an appropriate exercise regimen based on the types of activities you enjoy and your overall physical condition. If you have a diabetes-related complication, some exercises may contribute to further harm, so your program will also take into account your physical limitations. When you are ready to get started, you should begin slowly, and gradually build up your endurance and intensity over several weeks or months.

Exercise is very helpful in limiting weight gain and in keeping blood sugar levels from rising too high in women with gestational diabetes. However, pregnant women will want to avoid some of the more strenuous, high-impact exercises. Walking or swimming are both low-impact forms of exercise that can be beneficial.

Adopting a regular exercise program can enhance both your physical health and your mental outlook. All it takes is commitment and motivation. Whatever your exercise choice, be sure it's something you enjoy doing. There are many different kinds of exercises that you can try, so it should be easy to find an activity that you like and that is comfortable for you. Chapter 9 will discuss the many benefits—and the many types—of exercise in greater detail.

## MEDICATION

As you've already learned, insulin injections are a necessary factor in the treatment of type 1 diabetes. At this time, there simply is no other alternative. People with type 1 diabetes will die without insulin injections, because their bodies cannot produce insulin and therefore their cells cannot use glucose for energy.

Although type 2 diabetes has, in the past, been labeled non-insulin-dependent diabetes, it's estimated that some 30 to 40 percent of people with this type of diabetes need to take insulin. Treatment for type 2 diabetes depends upon the patient's fasting blood glucose levels and the presence of any diabetes-related health problems. Certain symptoms, such as hypertension or hyperlipidemia (elevated cholesterol and triglyceride levels), may require aggressive treatment even if blood glucose levels are not elevated. Some people may need insulin injections soon after an initial diagnosis of type 2 diabetes, especially if their blood sugar levels are very high at the time of diagnosis. However, after the insulin helps reduce blood glucose, a healthy diet and exercise program may be enough to keep blood sugar levels controlled without the need to continue treatment with insulin.

When a diet and exercise program is not sufficient, oral diabetes medications may be prescribed to help keep blood sugar levels within a target range. Some people with type 2 diabetes need a combination of insulin injections and oral diabetes medications to treat the condition. But remember that if you have type 2 diabetes and you need to take insulin or oral diabetes medications, it doesn't necessarily mean that your health is getting worse or that you're not doing a good management job on your own. And it also doesn't mean that you're going to have to continue taking insulin or other medications indefinitely. Adding medication to your treatment program may be only a temporary change.

It has been suggested that the longer you have type 2 diabetes, the more likely it is that you'll need insulin. Why? It's possible that over time your body may become more resistant to insulin, and chronic high blood glucose may add to the resistance. To make matters worse, age appears to cause a gradual decline in insulin production. So, keeping blood sugar levels under tight control seems to be the best way for people with type 2 diabetes to avoid having to take insulin injections. You should recognize, however, that for some people, this may be difficult or even impossible.

For gestational diabetes, dietary changes and special meal plans are often enough to regulate blood sugar levels, which must be closely monitored on a regular basis. Light or moderate exercise may also be recommended to help women with gestational diabetes control blood sugar. However, if gestational diabetes cannot be controlled with diet and exercise, then insulin treatments are necessary. (Oral medications should not be used by women who are pregnant or planning to become pregnant, because of the risk of birth defects.) Even though gestational diabetes is temporary, lasting only until the birth of the baby, it is a serious condition that can cause harm to the mother and her unborn child, so intensive treatment is necessary.

## OFFICE VISITS

Regularly scheduled checkups with members of your health-care team are a necessary part of your diabetes treatment program, regardless of the type of diabetes you have. Your primary-care physician will tell you how often you need to schedule office visits, although this recommendation may vary. As a general rule, if you take insulin for your diabetes or if you're having trouble controlling your glucose levels, you'll need to see your physician about every three months. Otherwise, you should see your doctor two or three times a year.

At certain times during the course of your treatment, you may need to visit your doctor more often (for example, if you are dealing with a diabetes-related complication). Also, if you are starting a new medicine or insulin program, or if your care plan has been adjusted, your doctor or other treatment-team members will advise you on how often you should check in. And, of course, if you are having trouble following your treatment program because of an illness—for example, if you've had nausea or vomiting that has made it difficult to eat properly, or if you've had a fever for more than a day—you should call your primary-care physician.

When you make your first appointment with your doctor, you should expect to have a complete physical examination. The doctor will take a medical history and run laboratory tests. Your later visits will not be as in-depth, although your doctor may order additional tests or refer you to a specialist if you appear to be developing a complication. During these follow-up appointments, your physician or another member of your treatment team will:

- Measure your height and weight.
- Take your blood pressure.

- Ask about any episodes of high or low blood sugar you've experienced.
- Ask if you've had difficulty following your treatment program.
- Check for symptoms of complications.
- Perform an $HbA1_c$ test.
- Check your cholesterol.
- Take a urine sample for testing.

Another important purpose of these visits is to review your treatment program to make sure you're meeting your goals. If you're having trouble managing your diabetes, then your doctor can make adjustments to your treatment program to help you establish better control.

### ADDITIONAL TREATMENT COMPONENTS

A truly complete diabetes treatment program will enable you to deal with the emotional aspects of living with diabetes—not just the physical difficulties. Stress management, for example, is an essential component in diabetes treatment, because emotional stress can cause major increases in your blood sugar levels, making your diabetes more difficult to control. To be successful in keeping your blood sugar levels controlled, you'll need to learn to handle stress well. In the long run, excessive levels of stress hormones are probably a major contributor to many diabetic complications. You'll learn some effective stress management techniques in chapter 24.

## Intensive Insulin Therapy

When you are first diagnosed with diabetes, the most important step you can take for your health is to begin a comprehensive treatment program. In chapter 5, you will learn how self-monitoring can help you bring your blood glucose down to your target level, and how keeping track of your test results will enable you to evaluate the efficacy of your diabetes care program. We have also touched upon the importance of maintaining a healthy eating plan, and of making regular exercise a part of your life—we'll return to these two facets of diabetes treatment in chapters 8 and 9. And so far this chapter has taught you all about using insulin to bring your blood sugar under control, whether you have type 1 or type 2 diabetes.

Now it's time to take a closer look at insulin therapy. Specifically, we will be discussing an approach known as *intensive insulin therapy.* The goal of this kind of treatment is to keep blood glucose under *tight control*—that is, to maintain blood sugar levels as near normal as possible by monitoring blood glucose several times during the day, and making adjustments in insulin based on food choices, exercise, and glucose test results. Intensive insulin therapy also involves keeping regular appointments with health-care professionals, and periodically reevaluating the prescribed diabetes treatment program. While this seems like a lot of work, studies have shown that this kind of intensive therapy can dramatically reduce the risk of developing diabetes-related complications, including eye problems, kidney disease, nerve disorders, cardiovascular disease, and foot and lower leg problems. Let's begin with a brief history of the landmark study that highlighted the benefits of tight control.

## THE DIABETES CONTROL AND COMPLICATIONS TRIAL

The Diabetes Control and Complications Trial (DCCT) was a ten-year study conducted by the National Institute of Diabetes and Digestive and Kidney Diseases that compared two approaches to managing diabetes: intensive and standard treatment. The primary goal of the study was to evaluate the effectiveness of intensive treatment on reducing the risk of diabetic complications. Researchers also measured the impact of tight control on managing the common complications of diabetes after they had already developed. More than 1,400 participants were involved in the DCCT.

To compare the efficacy of standard and intensive treatment, researchers divided the DCCT participants into two groups. The control group followed the standard diabetes treatment program: taking insulin once or twice a day at the same time each day, testing blood sugar levels once or twice daily, and meeting with a doctor or nurse approximately every three months. Participants in the intensive treatment group, on the other hand, learned how to adjust their insulin according to food intake and exercise, took insulin injections three or four times a day or used an insulin pump, and tested their blood sugar levels at least four times a day and once a week at three A.M. Individuals in the second group also followed a comprehensive diet and exercise program, and met with a health-care professional once a month. Their aim was to keep blood glucose levels between 70 and 120 mg/dl before meals and less than 180 mg/dl after meals, and to maintain an $HbA1_c$ of less than 6.05 percent.

The DCCT conclusively demonstrated that maintaining near-normal blood sugar levels can prevent, delay, or limit the severity of diabetes complications. The results of the study, published in 1994, showed that individuals with type 1 diabetes who maintained tight blood glucose control, with levels within a near-normal range, significantly reduced their chances of developing most of the major diabetes-related complications. Researchers reported that the normal risk of eye disease was reduced by 76 percent; the risk of nerve damage was reduced by 60 percent; the risk of kidney disease fell by 50 percent; and the risk of cardiovascular disease decreased by 35 percent.

All in all, the results of the DCCT were quite significant, and they offered much hope to individuals with diabetes hoping to avoid or minimize complications. However, intensive insulin therapy is not without its own problems. The most serious drawback is that tight control increases the risk of low blood sugar, or hypoglycemia. In fact, DCCT results showed that individuals in the intensive treatment group suffered three times as many hypoglycemic episodes as their counterparts in the standard group. Why did this happen? Overall blood glucose levels were kept within a lower range, and therefore it was easier for these levels to slip even lower.

Another unwanted effect of tight control was weight gain. Individuals in the intensive treatment group averaged a gain of ten pounds more than participants in the standard group. Whereas excess calories in the form of glucose had once spilled over into the urine, the extra glucose was stored in the body when tight control was achieved. And, as you'll remember from chapter 1, glucose that is not used for fuel is stored in the adipose (fat) tissues of the body.

## WHO BENEFITS FROM INTENSIVE INSULIN THERAPY?

Although all of the participants in the DCCT had type 1 diabetes, it seems safe to conclude that tight control can benefit people with other types of diabetes, as well. Intensive therapy is especially important for women with gestational diabetes, because keeping blood sugar levels within a near-normal range is so important to prevent complications of pregnancy and birth defects.

The main concern for people with type 2 diabetes seems to be the weight gain associated with tight control. Remember that obesity is one factor in the development of type 2 diabetes, and a primary goal for most people with this type of diabetes is weight loss. Experts warn that weight gain may be harmful for these individuals. But the fact remains that good control can really make a difference in future health, and people with type 2 diabetes should make every effort to keep their blood glucose levels within an acceptable range.

Not everyone is prepared to embark on the path to tight control, however. Some people are not as motivated to put in the effort that intensive therapy requires, preferring instead to remain at a level of moderate or even loose management. Others are concerned that intensive management will be more restrictive and impose more limitations in activities than standard treatment. In this case, the reverse seems to be true. Many people, in fact, enjoy greater flexibility as they become more adept at modifying their insulin doses to accommodate a variety of foods and other lifestyle factors, such as exercise.

Intensive management requires your energy and commitment. You'll need to learn the potential benefits and risks of keeping tighter blood glucose control, and to have a strong desire to improve your diabetes management skills. You will also have to work more closely with the members of your health-care team. Support from the significant people in your life—family, friends, and colleagues—is also an important factor in your success. Finally, be aware that intensive therapy carries a higher price tag, so you'll need to have the financial resources to undertake this kind of program.

Some people are not good candidates for intensive diabetes management. This treatment regimen is not recommended for older adults or for children under age thirteen. Also, individuals who have a history of frequent or severe hypoglycemic episodes, and those who experience hypoglycemia without warning symptoms, should probably not attempt this program. In addition, people with end-stage kidney disease, severe visual impairment, coronary artery disease, and other complications that have progressed to a more critical state are advised not to begin a program of intensive management. If you are interested in intensive therapy, talk to your doctor and other members of your health-care team to find out if you're a good candidate for this program.

## Some Final Treatment Notes

Becoming knowledgeable about diabetes and treatment for the disorder is an important part of learning to feel comfortable with self-management. There are numerous books available in bookstores and libraries that cover all aspects of living with diabetes. The American Diabetes Association is an excellent resource. To learn more about this organization, you can call (800) 342-2383 or (703) 549-1500, or visit *www.diabetes.org*. And remember the importance of maintaining open lines of communication with your health-care team. The members of your team are there for your support, and this includes answering any questions you may have about diabetes and diabetes treatment. Being informed and educated is the best way to start taking charge of your diabetes.

As important as treatment is, you cannot learn everything there is to know about diabetes self-management overnight. Learning is a *process*—it's not instantaneous. Take the time to learn as much as you can, recognizing that you can continue to refine and enhance your self-management skills.

The speed with which your treatment brings about results varies. Don't expect overnight success. However, with patience and proper adherence to a treatment program, you *can* and *will* experience improvement.

# PART TWO

# Changes in General Lifestyle

## CHAPTER FOUR

# Coping with Lifestyle Changes—An Introduction

So your life is going to change because of diabetes? Yes, that's all part of the package. But remember that throughout life, changes can occur for any number of reasons. If you begin a new job, you might have to wake up at a different time, commute in a new direction using a new form of transportation, or adjust to a different salary. And if your new job required you to move, you would have to learn your way around a new neighborhood.

In your case, it's diabetes that has now changed your life. Although you may think it will be impossible to ever lead a normal life again, this isn't necessarily true. However, it is vital to stop avoiding change, because the extent to which you now control your diabetes determines how healthy you will be in later years. Everybody has to make some lifestyle changes sooner or later, and many people find that they benefit from these changes. Because you have diabetes, you're going to benefit from good self-care because this will minimize or prevent complications in the future. So in your case, it's important to make changes that will help you make the most of your life right now—and even years from now.

To different degrees, diabetes can affect work, family life, sexual activity, social activity, finances, and other aspects of day-to-day living. Make up your mind to accept and work through any necessary changes. But also be aware that there are always things you can do to improve the way you live. In addition, remember that your lifestyle will, to a large degree, be of your own choosing. You'll automatically take many different factors into consideration when determining what you want you lifestyle to be.

You may decide to wait, to put things off—to avoid making any changes until you "feel better." But why wait? Why not try to see what you can do right now to improve the quality of your life, even while you're learning to live with diabetes?

## Making Changes

One very important part of coping with diabetes is learning to take control over as much of your life as possible. This means taking an active part in your treatment. As we've already discussed, controlling your diabetes requires time and effort. At first, you may feel a little overwhelmed at the thought of taking on the responsibilities of diabetes management. But realize that you will be helping yourself to feel better, and ensuring good health in the years to come. Focus on doing the best you can to help yourself.

A diagnosis of diabetes may seem totally negative. However, this diagnosis can be viewed as positive if it serves as motivation for change or self-improvement. You see, people change and grow not only when things are going well, but also during times of adversity. By looking at your life from a different perspective, you may be able to start weeding out those things that have not been good for you, and introducing better things.

## Getting Used to Changes

What are some of the factors that will determine how well you'll adapt to changes in your lifestyle? There are many. For example, what were you doing before you started experiencing symptoms of diabetes? How satisfied were you with your work and leisure activities? How supportive were the people close to you—both family and friends? How has your condition affected you, both physically and emotionally? These and other factors play a role in determining how you'll adjust to diabetes, its treatment, and any changes it necessitates. But that doesn't mean your hands are tied. You can improve the way you deal with virtually any factor.

The changes you'll make in your lifestyle because of diabetes require determination and self-discipline. At this point, your head may be spinning. You may fear that changes will have to be made in your activity schedule, your work, or your social life. You may also be apprehensive about dealing with physical discomfort and medication. You may even worry that you won't be able to perform your normal chores and responsibilities. These concerns are in no way unusual. Most people with diabetes do feel this way. But the fact that you can do much to improve your life should help you reduce your fears and approach change in a more positive way.

Some people with diabetes have difficulty making and adapting to changes in their lifestyles because of physical symptoms. For example, fatigue is a very common problem for individuals with diabetes. It can be caused by a single factor or a combination of different factors. As you've already learned, high or low blood glucose can certainly impact your energy levels, and weakness and fatigue are symptoms of both hypoglycemia and hyperglycemia. Maybe you've been pushing yourself too hard, trying to maintain the level of activity that was normal for you before your diagnosis of diabetes. And, believe it or not, you may feel fatigued even if you haven't been very active.

Additionally, consider the idea that you may feel tired or weak because of emotional problems. Many people who are depressed, angry, fearful, or anxious say that they feel fatigued. If you think that you may be tired and lethargic because of an emotional problem, try to pinpoint exactly what it is that's bothering you. Are you depressed because you've had to make some drastic changes in your lifestyle? Are you fearful that you won't ever adjust to living with diabetes? These are common concerns, and fortunately there are very real solutions that can help you cope with these concerns.

What's the best way to cope with fatigue? Rest. You see, fatigue can actually be a positive message—it's your body's ways of telling you that you need to slow down and stop pushing yourself. A good night's sleep or short naps during the day are great for coping with fatigue. Also, learn to prioritize! Focus on your top priorities when you have the energy, and leave less significant chores or activities for when you feel stronger. Set a schedule for yourself—try to avoid taking on too many strenuous activities in a row, and intersperse rest periods with any strenuous activities that you must follow through on.

## Guidelines for Change

As you begin to adjust to living with diabetes, remember that you don't have to go through this period of change alone. Your health-care team is there to help you develop a treatment plan that is appropriate for your needs. In developing your management program, you and your treatment team will consider a number of variables, including your age, daily schedule, responsibilities at work (or school) and at home, level of physical activity, eating habits, and social activities. This way, you can be sure that your diabetes management program will fit easily into your life, which will help minimize the lifestyle changes you'll have to make.

What happens if you decide not to make necessary lifestyle changes? This may indicate that you're trying to deny your situation. Denial is a very common coping strategy among people who are diagnosed with chronic conditions. But it's important to be aware of its negative side, too. What if denial keeps you from doing what you need to do? For example, what if you don't take your insulin, you don't eat properly, or you don't exercise? This is destructive denial, and it can hurt you. Hopefully, the fact you're reading this book in the first place shows that you're not really denying your condition. But continue to stay on top of this.

## As We Move On

Yes, you may have to make some changes in your lifestyle. But why assume that all of them will be negative? Isn't it possible that some of them will be for the better? Maybe you've been such a hard worker that you've never spent enough time with your family. If you have to cut back on your work schedule because of diabetes, perhaps you'll truly enjoy the increased time you'll be able to spend with your partner or children. Certainly, learning to take better care of yourself will pay off in the long run. So, as you modify your lifestyle, be sure to look for the positive.

CHAPTER FIVE

# Monitoring Your Blood Sugar Levels

Checking your blood sugar levels on a regular basis is one of the most important things you can do to keep your diabetes under control. Self-monitoring of blood glucose (SMBG) is an important and *necessary* part of diabetes management, regardless of the type of diabetes you have. Although SMBG may seem like a lot of work at first, it will be well worth the effort, because what you do today affects your future health and well-being. In the immediate future, you'll feel a whole lot better physically when you keep your blood sugar level within your target range. In the long run, you'll greatly reduce your risk of developing diabetes-related complications.

In 1994, the Diabetes Control and Complications Trial established a definite connection between blood glucose levels and the development of long-term complications. The DCCT conclusively demonstrated that maintaining near-normal blood sugar levels can prevent, delay, or limit the severity of diabetes complications. SMBG is an important part of "normalizing" glucose levels. By measuring your blood sugar levels every day, you'll be able to evaluate the efficacy of your diabetes treatment program. If you find that your blood sugar level is consistently above or below your target measurement, then you'll most likely need to work with your health-care team to adjust one or more factors involved in your treatment program.

Because no two people are exactly alike, there's no set formula that can tell you how your individual blood glucose level will respond to any number of factors. Think about this for a moment. Your blood sugar level is influenced by what you eat and how much you eat, the timing of your insulin or other medications, how active you are, your emotional state, and any physical stress that you may be experiencing, such as an illness. And these are only a few of the circumstances that will cause your blood sugar to rise or fall! That's why you need to know your levels—to become more familiar with how your body responds to these different factors so you can identify overall patterns in how your blood glucose level fluctuates.

## Choosing a Blood Glucose Monitor

When it comes to selecting a blood glucose monitor, you may feel a little at sea. Thanks to modern technology, there are many different products on the market that offer a variety of practical features. So how do you know which monitor is appropriate for your needs? You might start by checking with your doctor or diabetes educator to find out which monitors they recommend. Your pharmacist may also have some insight into which monitor best suits your individual needs. And you can always try asking someone who uses a glucose monitor about their satisfaction with a particular product.

The following considerations can help you weigh your options before you buy a blood glucose monitor.

- **How much does the monitor cost?** Price can be deceiving! Just because a monitor is expensive doesn't mean it's the best available. You can buy a high-quality monitor starting at under fifty dollars. Your goal is to find a product that has the features you need. Also, remember that you'll need additional supplies, such as test strips, that will add to the overall cost of your monitor.

Find out if your monitor and testing supplies are covered by your health insurance, and if so, get approval from your insurance company before you buy any product. Some companies offer full or partial funding for certain brands of monitors and supplies.

- **Is the monitor easy to use?** Some monitors are easier to use than others or require fewer steps in the testing procedure. If you have problems with your hands that will make the testing procedure difficult, you'll want to select a monitor that's easy to use. Your doctor, diabetes educator, or another member of your health-care team may be familiar with several different products, so it's a good idea to ask which brands they recommend.

- **Does the manufacturer offer customer assistance?** Most manufacturers of blood glucose monitors offer toll-free customer support. If you're having trouble using your monitor, you can call to ask for assistance at any time, twenty-four hours a day.

- **Does the monitor have a memory function?** Although it's strongly recommended that you write down the results of each blood glucose test, there may be times when you forget. If you think you won't be consistent in your record-keeping, you may want to invest in a glucose monitor that can store test results. However, remember that there's no substitute for keeping accurate daily records in a logbook or diabetes diary.

In addition to the standard blood glucose monitors available today, some brands offer special features for people who have physical problems that may make monitoring difficult. For example, if you have vision problems, you may want to select a monitor that displays large numbers. There are even some products that give verbal instructions to guide you through the testing procedure, and then audibly announce the test results.

# Goals for Blood Sugar Control

The results of the DCCT have proven that there is indeed a link between blood sugar control and the development of diabetes-related complications. Simply put, if you can consistently maintain good control of your blood sugar level, you will greatly reduce your risk of developing common complications. But what is "good control"?

Most people who have diabetes should aim to keep their blood glucose levels as close to normal as possible. However, there's a catch: Some individuals with diabetes are more prone to episodes of hypoglycemia, or low blood sugar, and it is appropriate for these people to keep their blood sugar levels a little higher than normal. Your doctor or diabetes educator can help you establish realistic goals for blood glucose control.

Table 5.1, below, presents recommended goals for blood glucose control. These recommendations have been adapted from publications of the American Diabetes Association and from other sources.

It's important to remember that you're trying to maintain *good* blood sugar control—you're not striving for perfection. Don't become too frus-

**TABLE 5.1. GOALS FOR BLOOD GLUCOSE CONTROL**

| TIME OF DAY | NORMAL | GOAL | WHEN TO TAKE ACTION |
|---|---|---|---|
| Before Meals | Less than 115 mg/dl | 80–120 mg/dl | If less than 80 mg/dl or over 140 mg/dl |
| Bedtime | Less than 120 mg/dl | 100–140 mg/dl | If less than 100 mg/dl or over 160 mg/dl |
| 1½–2 hours after meals | Less than 140 mg/dl | Less than 160 mg/dl | If more than 180 mg/dl |

trated if you don't achieve your target level every single time you check your blood sugar. Instead, continue to work with the members of your health-care team to determine more reasonable goals and to adjust your care plan so that you can reach those goals.

## Checking Your Blood Sugar Level

Blood glucose monitoring is a major component of your self-care program, so it's important that you test your blood sugar at the appropriate times, and that you take measures to get the most accurate results possible. Inaccurate results are useless to you because you will not be able to tell if you're effectively controlling your blood sugar levels.

To be sure you're getting correct test results, you should check your monitor's accuracy periodically. Your monitor should come with all of the supplies you will need to check for accuracy, including a control solution that is applied to one of the test strips. If the results with the control solution fall outside a specific range, then you'll know there's a problem with the monitor, the test strips, or both.

Always test your monitor for accuracy when you suspect an error in test results. The more experience you have with SMBG, the more you'll be able to anticipate your readings depending on the way you feel. If you think there's a discrepancy between your readings and the way you feel, you should also question your monitor's accuracy.

### HOW DO YOU CHECK BLOOD SUGAR?

Although blood glucose monitors vary in terms of cost and available features, the testing procedure is standard for all products. Before you begin, wash your hands with soap and warm water. This will help your blood vessels dilate, making it easier for you to get enough blood for the test.

All blood glucose monitors come with small needles called *lancets* that you will use to prick your finger and obtain a drop of blood. (You may think this is unpleasant at first; however, many people who have experience checking their blood sugar levels get so used to it they barely notice any discomfort at all!) The lancet is placed in a spring-loaded, pen-shaped lancing device that can be adjusted to control how deeply it pricks your finger. To obtain a drop of blood, put the device against your fingertip and release the spring. Any finger may be used to obtain the sample of blood.

The best way to minimize pain is to prick your finger quickly. Also, you may want to try using the side of your fingertip, rather than the middle, or "ball," of the fingertip. There are fewer nerve endings on the sides of the fingertips, so there should be less discomfort. Plus, if you prick the side of your fingertip, you will get a larger drop of blood. This is important, because one of the most common errors in blood glucose testing is failure to get a large enough drop of blood to sample.

## WHEN SHOULD YOU CHECK BLOOD SUGAR?

There's no hard-and-fast rule concerning how often you should check your blood sugar—it's really up to you and your health-care team to decide. Generally speaking, your schedule for monitoring your blood sugar is based on the type of diabetes you have, your goals for blood glucose control, and how you control your diabetes.

It's important to note that more frequent monitoring will enable you to see patterns in how your blood sugar level fluctuates, so you can work with your treatment team to adjust food intake, exercise, and medications accordingly. In short, the more often you check your blood sugar, the more you'll learn about your body's response to the factors that affect glucose levels, and the tighter your control becomes. And, of course, better control means reduced risk of complications.

### *Guidelines for Type 1 Diabetes*

In people with type 1 diabetes, blood glucose levels fluctuate constantly during the day. So, if you have this type of diabetes, your treatment goals determine how often you should check your blood sugar. If your aim is to keep your blood glucose level as close to a normal range as possible (70 to

120 mg/dl before meals, and less than 180 mg/dl after meals), then you'll need to test at least four to five times a day—before each meal, before bedtime, and in the middle of the night once a week. If your treatment program is less intensive—that is, if your goals are to prevent hyperglycemia and ketoacidosis—then you may only need to check your blood sugar twice a day.

Overall, the recommendation for blood glucose monitoring for type 1 diabetes is that you check as often as you're willing to. Your doctor will help you set up a monitoring schedule that will enable you to achieve your goals for blood glucose control. This schedule will also be based upon your lifestyle (for example, your work or school schedule) and how much you can afford to spend on supplies.

### *Guidelines for Type 2 Diabetes*

In people with type 2 diabetes, blood sugar levels tend to be more stable than they are in individuals with type 1 diabetes. However, if you are newly diagnosed with type 2 diabetes, your doctor will probably establish an intensive monitoring schedule at first, to help you get your blood sugar under control. This means that, like a person with type 1 diabetes, you'll need to check your blood sugar before meals, before bedtime, and in the middle of the night once a week. Once your blood sugar is consistently under good control, you will probably be okay checking your level once or twice daily. Again, your doctor will work with you to design a monitoring schedule that suits your needs.

If you have type 2 diabetes and you take insulin, you should check your blood sugar *at least* twice a day, although it's recommended that you check about four times a day. You will also need to measure your blood sugar more frequently any time a change is made in your treatment program.

## Recommendations for More Frequent Testing

There are some circumstances beyond your control that will make it necessary for you to check your blood sugar levels more often than your schedule dictates. Any of the following circumstances may make it necessary for you to check your blood sugar more frequently.

- When you're sick.
- If you suspect that your blood glucose levels are too high or too low.
- If you find that your blood glucose level is very high when you wake up in the morning.
- Whenever there's been a change in your treatment program.
- If you start taking a nondiabetic medication that can affect blood glucose levels.
- Before and after you exercise.
- If you experience frequent reactions to insulin.
- If you have lost or gained weight.
- If you are pregnant.
- When you try a new food.

All of the situations above can negatively impact your blood sugar level. By monitoring more often, you'll be certain to detect any changes in your blood sugar before a more serious problem develops.

## RECORDING YOUR TEST RESULTS

Every time you check your blood sugar level, write the results down in a self-care diary or notebook. This will enable you to see patterns in your blood glucose readings that provide clues about your diabetes control and to identify patterns that may be cause for concern. Then, if necessary, you and your health-care team can adjust one or more of the elements in your care plan accordingly, to get you back on the right track.

In addition to recording your test results, you should write down what you ate and how much you ate, since food has a direct effect on your blood sugar level. You should also jot down factors that may have affected your blood sugar levels, such as an illness, emotional stress, or strenuous physical activity.

A final word of caution: If you should recognize a pattern that indicates a need to adjust your treatment program, consult your doctor before making any changes. *Never* try to modify your diabetes care plan without the guidance of a health-care professional.

## Looking at the Big Picture

As you learned in chapter 2, the glycosylated hemoglobin ($HbA1_c$) test can be a very useful tool for measuring your average blood sugar level over a period of several weeks. Glucose in the bloodstream attaches to the hemoglobin on red blood cells, and the amount of glucose attached to the cells can be measured. Your body replaces red blood cells about every ninety days, so your $HbA1_c$ test results reflect your average blood glucose for approximately three months preceding the test. This is a better indicator of overall control than a one-time blood glucose test.

Glycosylated hemoglobin test results are given in the form of a percentage, indicating the percentage of hemoglobin molecules that are glycosylated. This percentage correlates with blood glucose values. For example, a score of 5 percent indicates an average blood glucose of 90 mg/dl. So what should your goal be? In general, people with diabetes should try to keep their $HbA1_c$ levels at about 7 percent or less.

The fructosamine test provides similar information to the $HbA1_c$ test. However, the fructosamine test measures how glucose is bound to proteins other than hemoglobin—proteins that do not have as long a life span as red blood cells. As a result, the test results reflect your average blood glucose for only two weeks. For this reason, the fructosamine test is not used as often as the $HbA1_c$ test as a measure of overall control.

## Moving on from Monitoring

In order to keep your diabetes under control, you must learn to recognize patterns in the rise and fall of your blood sugar level. This will enable you (with the supervision of your treatment team) to adjust other aspects of your diabetes care program to bring your blood glucose under control. As you will learn in the next several chapters, your ability to keep your blood sugar level within a target range depends on the interaction of a number of factors, including the type of medication you take, your diet, and your level of physical activity.

Self-monitoring of blood glucose is an essential first step in diabetes control. Remember, your goal is to successfully manage your diabetes so that you can lead a happy, healthy, and productive life.

# CHAPTER SIX

# Using Insulin

Like everything else in your diabetes management plan, it's important to balance each element to achieve success. In the past, doctors usually prescribed a single injection of insulin each day. Today, most doctors recommend multiple injections. Some people require two or three injections daily for best results. Your doctor will help you develop an insulin injection schedule that fits your lifestyle and that best helps control your diabetes.

Most people with diabetes fear the possibility of having to take insulin shots. Unfortunately, at present, insulin must be taken by injection or by pump in order to bring blood sugar levels down. Nevertheless, most people who take insulin report that the anticipation of taking insulin shots is much worse than actually taking the shots.

If you have type 1 diabetes, then you will have to give yourself daily insulin injections. This is not necessarily the case for type 2 diabetes; however, your doctor may tell you that you need to take insulin if you are unable to keep your blood sugar levels controlled with a balanced program of diet and exercise. Whatever the circumstance, you will doubtless have some concerns about giving yourself insulin shots. Never fear! The members of your treatment team will be there to show you the ropes, and to make sure you are comfortable using insulin.

# Insulin: A Review

Before we discuss the specifics of taking insulin shots to control blood sugar, let's take a moment to review insulin's functions in the body.

As you will remember from chapter 1, insulin is a hormone secreted by specialized cells in the pancreas called beta cells. Its primary function is to enable blood glucose, or blood sugar, to enter into the body's cells. Once inside the cells, the sugar molecules are used to produce the energy that's needed to keep the body running. Without insulin, glucose cannot be taken up by the cells, so it continues to circulate in the bloodstream rather than being used for fuel. As a result, the body becomes starved for energy.

If blood glucose is not used immediately by the body as fuel, insulin facilitates the transport of glucose to the liver and muscle tissues, where it is converted to glycogen for storage by the enzyme glycogen synthase. However, the capacity of the liver and muscle tissues to store glycogen is limited. If more carbohydrate is consumed than the body can use at that time, then some carbohydrate will be stored as fat in the adipose (fat) tissues. The body can call upon glycogen and fat reserves for energy during unanticipated fasts, or when extra energy is needed, such as during strenuous physical activity.

Besides its role in energy production, insulin is also important for the formation of muscle tissue. It increases protein synthesis by facilitating the transport of amino acids—the building blocks of proteins—to muscle cells. If insulin is insufficient, amino acids are not delivered to the muscle tissues, and as a result the muscles cannot develop properly. In fact, in the absence of insulin, muscles can become weak and may even atrophy.

People with type 1 diabetes have to take insulin injections each and every day because their bodies are not capable of producing insulin. Individuals with type 2 diabetes, on the other hand, do not necessarily require insulin shots, because their bodies are capable of producing insulin, although their body cells appear to be resistant to its effects. Women who have gestational diabetes require insulin only if they are unable to keep their blood sugar levels controlled with diet and mild exercise. However, gestational diabetes disappears after the birth of the baby, so continued treatment with insulin is not necessary.

## Sources of Insulin

In the past, beef insulin and pork insulin were the only varieties of insulin available to people with diabetes. As is obvious from their names, beef insulin comes from cows, while pork insulin comes from pigs. Today, many insulin-dependent individuals use human insulin instead of other animal products. Contrary to its name, human insulin does *not* come from human beings—it is manufactured in a laboratory. Synthetic human insulin is almost identical to the insulin that the human pancreas produces. It is considered superior to beef and pork insulin because it is absorbed faster and it has a shorter duration of action. Human insulin also produces fewer allergic or autoimmune reactions than the insulin that is extracted from animals, and it's usually less expensive.

## Types of Insulin

There are several different types of insulin available, which vary according to their action times. The *onset of action* refers to the length of time it takes the injected insulin to reach the bloodstream and to begin lowering blood glucose; the *peak of action* refers to the time during which the insulin is working at its maximum strength; and the *duration of action* refers to the overall length of time that the injected insulin continues to lower blood glucose. Keep in mind that each individual responds differently to insulin, so the action times of a particular type of insulin will vary from person to person. Factors such as injection site and technique of injection also influence how the injected insulin acts in the body. As you become more comfortable using insulin, you'll begin to learn how these different types of insulin will work for you.

There are four basic types of insulin, which are categorized according to their action times in the body. These are: rapid-acting insulin, regular or short-acting insulin, intermediate-acting insulin, and long-acting insulin.

## RAPID-ACTING INSULIN

There are currently two types of rapid-acting insulin available: *lispro* insulin (short for lysine-proline insulin) and *aspart* insulin. Rapid-acting insulin begins working very quickly within the body; the onset of action is between five and fifteen minutes. Therefore, this type of insulin must be taken directly before or after meals. Its peak of action is one to two hours, and its duration can last up to four hours.

## SHORT-ACTING INSULIN

The main type of short-acting insulin is *regular insulin.* Regular insulin—abbreviated with a capital R—is also called *clear insulin* because of its characteristic transparent appearance. This type of insulin begins working quickly in the body, usually within the half hour after injection. Its peak of action may last from one to three hours, and it is used up quickly by the body, within about five to seven hours. As a result, regular insulin must be injected several times during the day.

## INTERMEDIATE-ACTING INSULIN

Intermediate-acting insulin has a longer duration than short-acting insulin, but it takes more time to start working, and it also takes longer to reach its peak. This type of insulin begins working within two to four hours after injection, peaks between four and fourteen hours, and remains active for approximately twenty-four hours.

One type of intermediate-acting insulin is called *neutral protamine Hagedorn* (NPH), which is further abbreviated with a capital N. It contains a molecule known as a protamine, which reduces the speed of absorption by the body of the injected insulin. As a result, the insulin reaches the blood more slowly and has a longer peak and duration. An advantage of intermediate-acting insulin's slower action time is that fewer insulin injections are required each day.

Some people are allergic to the protamine in NPH. These individuals often respond better to another intermediate-acting insulin called *Lente* (abbreviated with a capital L). The name Lente comes from the Latin for "slow." This type of insulin works more slowly because it has added zinc.

Both types of intermediate-acting insulin are recognizable by their characteristic cloudy appearance.

### LONG-ACTING INSULIN

*Ultralente* is the only type of long-acting insulin available. This type of insulin takes approximately four to six hours to begin lowering blood glucose, and its peak of action lasts from eight to twelve hours or more. Long-acting insulin has a duration of action of up to thirty-six hours, so it can provide an almost continuous insulin release. However, most people who use ultralente insulin combine it with a short-acting insulin, often used at mealtimes.

## Mixing Different Types of Insulin

You may find that mixing different types of insulin is the best way to keep your blood sugar controlled. Usually, short-acting insulin (R) and intermediate-acting insulin (N) are mixed together. The actions of the two types of insulin complement each other: As the short-acting insulin wears off after about six hours, the intermediate-acting insulin begins to peak, and continues to work in the body for eighteen to twenty-four hours.

Premixed insulins are available for people who use a mixture of intermediate- and short-acting insulins. The most common mixture is 70 percent N and 30 percent R. There are also mixtures of 50 percent N and 50 percent R available. These premixed preparations are helpful for individuals who have trouble mixing the insulins themselves because of poor eyesight or problems with their hands. They are also more convenient for people who have stabilized their blood sugar levels with the 70/30 or 50/50 intermediate- and short-acting mixtures.

If you decide to mix your own insulin, there are a few things you need to know:

- Keep the two types of insulin separated; avoid injecting one type of insulin into a bottle that contains a different type
- Don't mix different brands of insulin
- Use mixed preparations of N and R insulin immediately or store the mixture in the refrigerator until you are ready to use it
- Don't mix any other medication with your insulin

## Concentrations of Insulin

The strength of insulin is measured according to its *concentration.* The concentration of insulin is the number of units of insulin dissolved in a specific volume of fluid. For example, a common concentration is U-100, which means that there are 100 units of insulin per one milliliter of fluid. These days, the strength of insulin is standardized; in the past, there were many different concentrations available, which added to the confusion of knowing how much to take.

Most of the insulin sold in the United States has a concentration of U-100. There are also more concentrated forms available, such as U-500 (500 units of insulin per milliliter of fluid), which are used less frequently. Insulin that has a strength of U-500 is generally only prescribed for people who have severe insulin resistance. A more dilute concentration, U-40, is no longer used in the United States, but it is still available in Europe and in Latin America, so you need to be especially careful if you travel to those areas.

## Buying and Storing Insulin

When it comes to buying insulin, it does pay to shop around for the best price for the insulin you need. Prices can vary by several dollars a bottle depending on where they're sold. Still, be sure to purchase your insulin from a reputable pharmacy so you can be assured that the product is of good quality. Also, it's important to develop a relationship with your pharmacist—make sure that he or she will take an interest in your medical needs, and will be available to answer any questions you might have about your insulin. You'll probably be in contact with this person a lot over the years.

Always check the expiration date on the insulin bottle before you buy the product. You should not buy or use any insulin after its expiration date has passed. If you decide to buy more than one bottle at a time, keep in mind your needs—will you use the entire quantity that you purchase before the expiration date? And keep your eyes and ears open in case there's news of a product recall (although this happens very rarely). Check the control number on each of your bottles to see if it matches that of the recalled lot.

Insulin can be stored at room temperature or in the refrigerator—it's a matter of personal choice. Manufacturers often recommend keeping insulin in the refrigerator, because it will stay potent for a longer period of time. However, cold insulin may make the insulin shot more painful. For this reason, many doctors recommend storing the insulin at room temperature, even though it won't last as long. In general, an unopened bottle of insulin kept at room temperature will last for about one month; stored in the refrigerator, it will last about three months. If you decide to keep your insulin in the refrigerator, you can warm it up after it has been drawn into the syringe—just roll the syringe gently back and forth in your hands.

Insulin is a fragile protein, and it must be handled with care. Do not store your insulin at extreme temperatures. If the insulin gets too cold, it can clump or freeze; if it gets too hot, it can spoil. The best rule to remember is this: If the temperature is comfortable for you, it will probably be safe for your insulin.

## Buying Syringes

Insulin syringes are available in different sizes. The largest insulin syringes hold up to 100 units (one milliliter) of insulin. Others hold 25, 30, or 50 units of insulin. Make sure that the syringes you buy are large enough to hold your entire dose of insulin. For example, if your doctor has prescribed 40 units of insulin, you'll need to buy syringes that hold at least 50 units each.

It's very important to check the markings on the syringes you choose. Some syringes have a mark for each unit, while others have a mark for every two units. Additionally, each syringe should be marked with the number of units it holds.

## Instructions for Injecting Insulin

It's perfectly natural to feel anxious the first few times you give yourself insulin injections. You may be worried that the shot will hurt, or that you won't be able to draw up the right dose. Or you may feel apprehensive about fitting insulin shots into your daily schedule. But there are millions of people with diabetes out there who have mastered insulin injections—they're proof that the procedure can be quick and relatively painless. And if so many others have effectively made insulin injections a part of their daily routines, there's no reason why you can't have the same success.

### DRAWING UP A SINGLE TYPE OF INSULIN

Your doctor or certified diabetes educator will teach you how to give yourself insulin injections. Technique is very important in order to make sure the insulin is being delivered properly and safely. Don't be afraid—you'll have plenty of opportunities to practice before you begin giving yourself injections without supervision.

You can use the following steps as a reference when you give yourself insulin shots. But be sure to ask your doctor or diabetes educator any specific questions you have about your insulin injections.

1. Wash your hands.
2. Gather your equipment together. You'll need a bottle of insulin, an insulin syringe, and an alcohol swab, or alcohol and cotton balls.
3. Check the bottle of insulin for cracks and leaks. Make sure the insulin has not passed its expiration date. Always check the insulin's appearance before using it. Short-acting Insulin (Regular) should be clear—don't use the insulin if it looks cloudy, or if you notice floating particles or color changes, which may suggest that the insulin has lost its strength or is contaminated. Intermediate-acting and long-acting insulin should be uniformly cloudy (the appearance should be similar to skim milk) after they are mixed. Do not use these products if they are not uniformly cloudy, or if you see clumps of insulin in the liquid or sticking to the bottom or sides of the bottle.
4. Gently roll the insulin bottle between the palms of your hands so the contents are equally distributed throughout the solution. Don't shake your insulin—shaking creates air bubbles.
5. Remove and discard the colored cap of the bottle; leave the rubber stopper and metal band in place. Clean the bottle top with an alcohol swab and allow the top to dry.
6. Pull back the plunger of the syringe so that the syringe fills with air. The amount of air you draw into the syringe should equal the appropriate number of units for your dosage.
7. Take the cap off the needle. Insert the needle into the bottle of insulin through the rubber stopper. Push down on the plunger and inject the air into the bottle.
8. Keeping the needle inside the bottle of insulin, turn both the bottle and the syringe upside down. Hold the bottle with one hand. With the other hand, draw back the plunger to the desired dose. The end of the plunger should be exactly on the mark for your dose. Don't remove the needle just yet.

9. Look at the insulin in the syringe. Do you see any air bubbles? If you find air bubbles, gently tap on the syringe until the bubbles float up to the top; then, slowly push the plunger down to "inject" the insulin back into the bottle. Draw the plunger back to your dose. You may have to repeat this step a few times to get rid of all the air bubbles.
10. Before you remove the needle from the bottle, make sure that you have withdrawn the correct dose. Then pull the needle out of the rubber stopper. Recap the needle if you need to put the syringe down or if it will be a while before you give yourself the injection.

## CHOOSING AN INJECTION SITE

Insulin is injected into the fatty tissue just under the skin, rather than directly into the bloodstream. The abdomen is usually the best area for an insulin injection. The top and outer parts of the thighs are also commonly used injection sites; this is best done when you're sitting down. Other good sites are the buttocks, the hips, and the backs of the upper arms. Do not give yourself injections in the two-inch area around your navel, in the groin or inner thigh area, or near scars or stretch marks.

Be aware that insulin is absorbed at different rates by different areas of the body. This must be taken into consideration in your treatment routine. Insulin is absorbed most quickly when injected into the abdomen; more slowly when injected into the arms; and even more slowly when injected into the thighs or buttocks. Other factors that affect the rate of absorption include: the type of insulin, the depth of the injection, and even the temperature of the skin and the air surrounding the skin.

You should rotate injection sites to avoid overusing a particular site. Some people randomly choose different sites of the body, while others may rotate within one general body area. If you are staying within the same general area, try to space your injection sites about one-inch apart (approximately the width of a finger). Make sure you have a way to remember the site of your previous injection.

If you are planning to exercise, don't give yourself an injection in the area that you will be exercising. For example, if you're going to go running, you shouldn't inject your insulin into your thighs. Insulin is absorbed faster due to increased circulation, and this can cause hypoglycemia.

## GIVING YOURSELF AN INSULIN INJECTION

Again, your doctor or diabetes educator will work closely with you until you feel comfortable giving yourself insulin injections without supervision. If you're still a little nervous, you can refer to the following instructions. But remember to ask a member of your treatment team any specific questions you have about insulin injections.

1. Choose your injection site. Clean the site with an alcohol swab or soap and water.
2. With your nondominant hand, pinch up about an inch of skin.
3. Hold the syringe like a dart. Quickly push the needle into the pinched-up skin at a 90-degree angle. If you are thin, you may want to insert the needle at an angle that's closer to 45 degrees. Do not insert the needle at an angle that's less than 45 degrees.
4. Still holding the skin pinched up, push the plunger all the way down to inject the insulin.
5. Pull the needle straight out after all of the insulin is injected. Cover the injection site with an alcohol pad, and release the pinched-up skin.
6. Place the cover back on the needle, and dispose of the syringe.

If you see blood around the injection site, gently apply pressure on the site for a minute or two. *Do not rub the injection site*—this may cause the insulin to be absorbed too quickly.

## DISPOSING OF THE SYRINGE

Because syringes and lancets come in contact with human blood, they are considered to be—*and must be discarded as*—medical waste. It is illegal to throw out used needles with everyday trash. Check with your sanitation company to find out how to dispose of used needles and medical wastes.

It's also a good idea to find out if your local health department, pharmacy, or hospital has a syringe disposal service.

After you have used a syringe, put it in an opaque, puncture-proof container, such as the kind that contains bleach or laundry detergent. You can also use an empty coffee can with a small hole cut in the plastic lid. *Do not recycle* any containers that you use to dispose of your syringes.

To save money, you may be tempted to reuse a disposable needle and syringe. If you clean and maintain the syringe properly, it is okay to reuse the syringe under some circumstances. However, disposable syringes purchased in quantity can be an inexpensive insurance that there won't be any problem. But you should always remember this important rule: *Never* use another person's syringe, and *never* let anyone else use yours.

## Side Effects of Insulin

The most common side effect of insulin shots is low blood sugar, or hypoglycemia, which is sometimes called an *insulin reaction.* This condition usually results from too much insulin, although it can also occur due to delaying or skipping a meal, or exercising too hard or for too long. Warning signs of hypoglycemia include fatigue, hunger, confusion, and shakiness. If blood sugar drops too low, unconsciousness or seizures may result.

Hypoglycemia can usually be prevented if you take your medication at regular times and plan your meals in conjunction with insulin action. However, should you experience any of the warning signs of hypoglycemia, it's important to eat or drink a high-sugar snack or beverage to quickly bring your blood sugar back up to a safe level. You should also make sure that your family, friends, and coworkers know what to do if you're unable to help yourself. Chapter 10 discusses the symptoms of and treatment for hypoglycemia in greater detail.

Some people experience local skin reactions to insulin, although this is relatively rare. *Lipoatrophy* is caused by the loss of fatty tissue under the skin. This usually appears as little dents under the skin at the injection site; the site may also appear slightly depressed and feel firm to the touch. Experts believe that lipoatrophy is caused by an immune reaction to insulin, although it's also possible that the reaction results from repeated trauma to the skin in one spot. The chances of having an adverse reaction to insulin are probably greater with the use of beef or pork insulin, because the immune system is more likely to interpret the insulin as a foreign substance. Using human insulin and rotating injection sites are the best ways to avoid or alleviate lipoatrophy.

*Hypertrophy* is another skin reaction that may result from insulin injections. This condition results from an accumulation of fat cells at the injection site that looks similar to scar tissue, and may cause the skin to appear lumpy. The affected area feels soft to the touch and should not be painful or uncomfortable. Hypertrophy can be avoided by frequently rotating injection sites.

Allergic reactions to insulin generally appear as itching, redness, and pain at the injection site. Groups of small bumps that look like hives may also result. These irritations usually clear up on their own; however, you should report any unusual reactions to insulin to your doctor.

## Modern Methods for Insulin Administration

Thanks to extensive research, there are a number of revolutionary insulin delivery devices available to people with diabetes. Insulin pumps and pens have made insulin therapy a whole lot more convenient for individuals who are always on the go. And jet injectors seem to have taken the sting out of injections for "needle phobics." But who are the best candidates for these advanced devices? Read on to find out.

### INSULIN PUMPS

Insulin pumps are computerized devices that deliver insulin at a slow, continuous rate throughout the day. The pump resembles a pager, and it can be worn on your belt or in your pocket. A measured amount of insulin is pumped through flexible plastic tubing to a small needle inserted just under the skin and taped in place. This type of insulin delivery is called continuous subcutaneous (under the skin) insulin infusion, or CSII for short.

The pump is programmed to deliver a steady quantity of insulin, known as a *basal dose,* twenty-four hours a day. Before meals, a larger amount, or *bolus dose,* is delivered at the touch of a button to compensate for rising blood sugar caused by food intake. If you decide to use a pump to take your insulin, your doctor will determine your basal and bolus doses.

Insulin pumps offer several advantages over syringes for insulin delivery. For one thing, most people who use insulin pumps are able to gain greater blood glucose control, which reduces their risk of developing diabetes-related complications. Pumps are also more convenient. There's no need to take time out to fill syringes and take insulin shots—pumps hold a one- to two-day supply that is delivered continuously, day and night.

Be aware that insulin pumps are not appropriate for everyone. If you are considering making the switch, you should know that you'll have to measure your blood glucose levels more frequently, because this kind of intensive insulin therapy carries with it an increased risk of hypoglycemia. You will also have to be patient—it will take some time to learn what basal dose works best for you, when you'll need to adjust your basal dose, and how big a bolus dose you should take before each meal. It's also important to have good support from your health-care team.

## INSULIN PENS

Insulin pens are compact, convenient devices that are especially useful for people who are on the go. Each pen holds a premeasured cartridge filled with Regular, NPH, or 70/30 premixed insulin; the dosage is set by turning a dial in one- or two-unit increments. All you have to do is screw a capped needle onto the end of the pen and set the dose. Because the pen is so small and lightweight, it's discreet and easy to carry, and its all-in-one design makes it easy to use for people whose coordination is impaired. A major drawback, however, is price—insulin pens cost up to twice as much per unit of insulin compared with standard vials.

### JET INJECTORS

Some people with diabetes prefer to use jet injectors, rather than syringes with needles. The jet injector releases a very fine jet stream of insulin that pierces the skin—no needles are involved, so it seems to be the ideal choice for people who are "needle-phobic." However, jet injectors are not for everyone with diabetes. If you decide to try using this device, be aware that you'll need to receive thorough training, because incorrect use can cause bruising and even scarring. Also, jet injectors can be expensive, so you should check to make sure your insurance covers the purchase.

## What Does the Future Hold?

Pancreas transplantation is one of the new methods being investigated, and the findings have sometimes been miraculous. Part or all of a new pancreas (from a living relative or from someone who has died) is surgically implanted in the pelvic area. The old pancreas remains in place—it still produces digestive enzymes even though it doesn't produce insulin. In some cases, individuals who have received successful pancreas transplants may not need to take insulin anymore and may have normal blood glucose levels. In addition, successful transplant recipients have noticed many diabetes side effects being minimized or eliminated, and complications being further delayed or prevented.

The problem with pancreas transplantation is the same as for any organ transplant. The body perceives it as a foreign entity, and the immune system attacks it. As a result, in order for it to remain a viable part of the body, people receiving pancreas transplants must receive powerful immunosuppressant drugs so that rejection does not take place. These drugs, designed to prevent the immune system from rejecting the new pancreas, can also lower resistance to other diseases.

Research is also being done with the idea of transplanting islet cells (the cells that produce the insulin) rather than the whole pancreas. It is believed that islet cell transplantation would be less dangerous than transplating the whole pancreas. However, this is even more experimental than pancreas transplantation, because it is still not known exactly how many islet cells are needed, where they should be placed in the body, and what kind of treatment is necessary to minimize the chances of rejection.

## Give It Your Best Shot

If you're afraid of giving yourself insulin injections, take heart. There's no reason why you can't learn how to manage this aspect of your diabetes care—especially with the strong support of your treatment team. Learning how to give yourself injections takes time and patience. But isn't it worth the effort? After all, you're ensuring your present and future health.

CHAPTER SEVEN

# Taking Oral Diabetes Medications

Oral diabetes medications are prescription drugs that can help your body use the glucose from food for energy. These drugs can help you keep your blood sugar under control only if they are used as an integral part of your diabetes care plan, which also includes a healthy diet, regular exercise, and daily blood glucose monitoring.

## When Are Oral Diabetes Medications Prescribed?

The first course of action for anyone who is diagnosed with type 2 diabetes is to start a personalized diet and exercise program to bring blood sugar under control. For some people, a balanced diet and regular exercise are all that's needed to control their diabetes. However, you may find that diet and exercise alone are just not enough to keep your blood sugar within a target range. In this case, the answer may be medication.

Oral diabetes medications will not help everyone with type 2 diabetes. They are more likely to work in certain cases, such as for those who have had high blood glucose for less than ten years, who are either of normal weight or somewhat obese and who are able and willing to consistently follow a healthy meal plan, and who have some insulin secreted by their pancreas. In people who are very thin, the drugs tend to work less effectively. In general, these drugs are not used for people with type 1 diabetes. However, there are some people with type 1 diabetes who may benefit from certain oral medications in addition to their insulin program.

Oral diabetes medications are *not* insulin, and should not be used by people with type 1 diabetes, whose bodies are unable to produce insulin. Instead, these medications work with the insulin that the body does produce to keep blood sugar under control. In general, oral medications work well for people who:

- Developed diabetes after the age of forty.
- Have had diabetes for less than five years.
- Are of normal weight.
- Have never used insulin or have taken only 40 units or less of insulin a day.

Pregnant women and women who are breast-feeding should *not* take oral medications for blood sugar control, because the effects of these medications on unborn children and on newborns are not yet known.

## Types of Oral Diabetes Medications

There are five classes of medications available for the treatment of diabetes. Some work by stimulating the pancreas to produce more insulin; some increase the amount of glucose taken up by the muscles; and some slow the rate at which glucose is absorbed by the digestive system. The different types of medications are:

- Sulfonylureas.
- Biguanides.

- Alpha-glucosidase inhibitors.
- Thiazolidinediones.
- Meglitinides.

Now let's take a closer look at the medications available for the treatment of type 2 diabetes.

## SULFONYLUREA DRUGS

Sulfonylureas were the only oral medications used to treat diabetes in the United States until 1994, and most oral medications available today fall into this category. These drugs work by stimulating the pancreas to produce more insulin so that more glucose can be taken up by the body's cells. Sulfonylureas also lower blood glucose by improving insulin sensitivity and decreasing glycogen breakdown for glucose in the liver.

Currently there are a number of different types of sulfonylurea drugs prescribed in the United States, including:

- Tolazamide (Tolinase).
- Glipizide (Glucotrol).
- Glimepiride (Amaryl).
- Glyburide (Diabeta, Micronase).

Medications such as tolbutamide (Orinase), acetohexamide (Dymelor), and chlorpropamide (Diabinese) are other examples of sulfonylureas; however, these drugs are not commonly prescribed nowadays.

Individuals whose bodies are no longer able to produce insulin should not use sulfonylureas. Also, people with liver or kidney disease should not take these medications. Individuals who take sulfonylurea drugs are advised to minimize their alcohol intake, because drinking alcohol increases the risk of hypoglycemia.

The most serious side effect caused by sulfonylureas is low blood sugar, which can be severe and may last beyond the time of the drug's effectiveness. Other adverse effects include gastrointestinal upset, loss of appetite, skin rashes, and itching. Some sulfonylurea drugs, such as chlorpropamide, may cause water retention, with symptoms including headache, nausea, drowsiness and, in the most extreme cases, convulsions. If you find that you are experiencing any uncomfortable side effects—no matter how minor—from taking sulfonylureas, let your doctor know. He or she can prescribe a different medication that may be less likely to cause these problems.

## BIGUANIDES

Biguanides help people with type 2 diabetes in a different way than the sulfonylureas. Rather than stimulating the pancreas to secrete more insulin, this type of medication lowers blood glucose levels by decreasing glucose production by the liver. It also improves insulin action, and reduces the amount of glucose from food that is absorbed by the small intestine. At this time, the main biguanide medication is metformin (Glucophage).

It is estimated that 80 percent of people who try metformin benefit from it. This makes it extremely effective, especially for individuals who do not benefit from sulfonylureas. Metformin offers other potential benefits, aside from its obvious glucose-lowering action in the body. There is practically no risk of hypoglycemia with this medication, unless it is taken in combination with other glucose-lowering agents, such as insulin or sulfonylureas. Physicians have observed that this medication can help lower high blood levels of triglycerides and the "bad" low-density lipoprotein (LDL) cholesterol in their patients. And metformin appears to cause weight loss in many people who take it.

The use of metformin may cause abdominal bloating, diarrhea, loss of appetite, and nausea and vomiting. Some people who use metformin have also reported that the medication leaves a metallic taste in the mouth. However, these problems are usually temporary, and disappear as the body adjusts to the medication.

Individuals who have suffered a heart attack or who have severe chest and heart trouble are advised not to use this drug. Additionally, metformin should not be given to heavy drinkers.

Metformin may cause a rare but serious condition known as *lactic aci-*

*dosis,* in which lactic acid enters the bloodstream quickly, changing the acid level of the body. People who have liver or kidney problems are more likely to develop lactic acidosis, and so should not take this medication. Alcohol can increase the risk of this condition, so people who take metformin should avoid the use of alcohol. Symptoms of lactic acidosis include weakness, tiredness, muscle pain, trouble breathing, coldness, dizziness, and irregular heartbeat.

## ALPHA-GLUCOSIDASE INHIBITORS

Alpha-glucosidase inhibitors are medications that work in the small intestine by temporarily blocking the action of certain enzymes necessary for the digestion of some carbohydrates. These medications must be taken shortly before or with meals to reduce the high peak of glucose that occurs after food is eaten. Types of alpha-glucosidase inhibitors include acarbose (Precose, Prandase) and miglitol (Glyset).

Alpha-glucosidase is probably best suited as a single drug for people who have relatively mild type 2 diabetes. The medication may also be combined with other glucose-lowering agents such as sulfonylureas. However, be aware that combining alpha-glucosidase inhibitors with other medications increases the risk of hypoglycemia; the use of alpha-glucosidase inhibitors alone will not have this effect. Should hypoglycemia occur, it is best treated with glucose or lactose (milk sugar), since acarbose and miglitol slow the absorption of some carbohydrates such as sucrose (table sugar).

Side effects caused by the use of alpha-glucosidase inhibitors can include gastrointestinal discomfort such as gas and diarrhea. Starting with a low dose and gradually increasing the dose until the target level is reached can prevent the occurrence of side effects. Adverse effects usually disappear within three to four weeks, as the body becomes more accustomed to the medication. Individuals with chronic intestinal or liver problems should not take alpha-glucosidase inhibitors.

## THIAZOLIDINEDIONES

Rosiglitazone (Avandia) and pioglitazone (Actos) are medications in the thiazolidinedione class. These drugs work by decreasing insulin resistance, and by increasing the uptake of glucose by muscle and fat cells. They also help decrease glucose production by the liver. Thiazolidinediones should be taken once a day, and do not necessarily have to be taken with food.

Individuals with mild type 2 diabetes are most likely to benefit from the use of thiazolidinediones. Also, there is some evidence that people with type 1 diabetes may be able to reduce their insulin dosage by using a drug from this class in combination with insulin. Used by themselves, thiazolidinediones are not likely to cause hypoglycemia; however, when used in combination with insulin or sulfonylureas, the risk of hypoglycemia increases.

The thiazolidinediones offer some potential benefits beyond their glucose-lowering action. They may reduce blood levels of triglycerides and "bad" low density lipoprotein (LDL) cholesterol. Some patients have even reported weight loss after starting therapy with thiazolidinediones. Recent research has shown an increased effectiveness of blood glucose control when drugs from this class are used in conjunction with metformin.

Few side effects have been reported with the use of thiazolidinediones. However, use of these medications should be avoided by people with liver disease, and should be used with caution in patients with heart problems.

Another drug in this class, Troglitazone (Rezulin), was removed from the market by the FDA because it caused severe liver damage in a number of the individuals taking the drug.

## MEGLITINIDES

A medication known as repaglinide (Prandin), the first drug developed and approved in the meglitinide category, can be used to manage the rise in blood glucose that occurs after meals. Repaglinide works by binding to sites on the beta cells of the pancreas, which stimulates the pancreas to secrete more insulin. This medication has a quick onset and short duration of action that is concentrated around the mealtime glucose load. It must be taken with meals to control blood glucose effectively. If a meal is skipped, so is the medication; if a meal is added during the day, an extra tablet should be taken before the meal. Repaglinide may be used in combination with metformin.

As with sulfonylureas, repaglinide can cause blood sugar levels to drop too low, resulting in hypoglycemia. This drug also slightly increases the risk of cardiovascular problems when compared with other oral diabetes medications. Side effects include sinus and respiratory problems. Antibacterial drugs, antifungal drugs, and troglitazone can interact with this medication.

## Choosing the Appropriate Medication

How does your physician determine which medication will work best for you? Many factors must be taken into account, including: your age and overall health, the type of diabetes you have, the severity of your diabetes, how much your blood sugar fluctuates, and any diabetes-related symptoms or complications you're experiencing. Of course, it's important for you to inform your doctor about any other medications—prescription or over-the-counter—that you are currently taking or considering taking. Some prescription and OTC drugs can interact with certain oral diabetes medications, and can substantially reduce the benefits of the oral medications. Certain drug interactions may even be dangerous.

Some amount of trial and error may be necessary to determine the medication and proper dosage that will suit your needs. This is not unusual, even after all of the facts are considered. Lots of people have to try different kinds of diabetes medications in order to find the combination that works best for them. This may be very frustrating, but the results are worthwhile. Make sure you understand exactly why you're taking the medication and what it's supposed to do.

## Additional Medication 'Minders

Because of the chemical natures of oral diabetes medications and the way they may interact in your body, it's extremely important that you follow your doctor's orders when taking the drugs prescribed for you. Follow your doctor's prescription as carefully as possible. *Never* mix drugs without knowing if the combination is safe. If you need to take many different pills, make sure that you don't play with your dosage, or with the times you take them, or move around the number of pills you take at a particular time.

Once you've begun a medication program, make sure you let your physician know how effective the drugs are in helping you with your condition. Any significant changes in your health, good or bad, should be reported to your treatment team.

It is almost impossible for any physician to keep up with all the thousands of different types of prescription drugs on the market. However, this is the pharmacist's specialty. Frequently, pharmacists know even more than physicians as far as what drugs can go together and what drugs interact dangerously. So it can be very helpful for you to develop a good working relationship with your local pharmacist. Not only will your pharmacist be able to tell you about the medication that has been prescribed for you, but he may be able to help you reduce costs. Occasionally, generic products that cost less than their brand-name counterparts may be available. However, in some individuals the generic drug will not work as well as the brand-name medication. If you have a good relationship with your pharmacist, you will find it a lot easier to get the medication you need.

## A Prescription for Good Control

By the time you read this book, there may be additional drugs on the market that are far superior to the ones you've been taking. There is nothing wrong with discussing your medication with your treatment team and asking if new drugs are available. But remember, this doesn't mean that these will necessarily be better for you.

This chapter doesn't include all medications used by people with diabetes. Instead, it emphasizes the more common ones. But at least this information will help you become more familiar with the ones you may hear about. So if your doctor prescribes something new, ask about it. Then, if your new medication makes you feel better, you'll know why!

CHAPTER EIGHT

# Following Your Meal Plan

Food, glorious food! Do you like to eat? Eating is one of the great pleasures of life, so you may be upset by the realization that you'll have to make some changes in your diet and eating habits. A proper eating plan is essential to the success of any diabetes treatment program, and—as you'll discover in this chapter—what you eat, how much you eat, and when you eat are crucial factors in controlling your diabetes. The more you are dedicated to adopting a balanced, nutritious diet, the better you'll be able to control your diabetes and, believe it or not, the more you'll be able to enjoy eating.

It *is* possible to make a healthful eating a part of your overall diabetes treatment program—millions of people with diabetes have proven that. So read on! There's a lot of good news ahead.

## Goals for Your Diet

When you first undertake a treatment program, you'll need to learn how to modify your diet and eating habits in order to manage your diabetes. Your dietitian will assess your nutritional status and work with you to develop a personalized diet plan. And, together with you physician and other members of your health-care team, your dietitian will help you to determine how to balance your eating plan with your other treatment requirements, such as exercise and medication.

Your diet plan should be developed with specific goals in mind. In 1994, the American Diabetes Association revised its nutritional recommendations, based on the idea that no single dietary approach will work for everyone. The new approach, which is more flexible than the earlier guidelines, includes the following recommendations:

- Maintain blood glucose levels as close to normal as possible.
- Attain and maintain a reasonable weight.
- Achieve healthy blood cholesterol and triglyceride levels.
- Minimize or prevent short-term complications, such as hyperglycemia and hypoglycemia, and long-term complications, including kidney disease, cardiovascular disease, and nerve damage.
- Improve overall health through optimal nutrition.

There are many factors that you and your dietitian must take into consideration in order to design a diet plan that will be most effective for you. These include how many calories you need to take in, your food preferences, seasonings that you like, your traditions, your ethnicity, and your social eating patterns, among others. Your daily diet should contain a healthy balance of fats, proteins, and carbohydrates, and should also include a nice variety of tasty foods that you enjoy. This increases the likelihood that you will stick with your dietary program. All of your unique needs will be taken into consideration in developing your eating plan. Don't think of this as a diet; it's a program that will enable you to take charge of your diabetes and improve the quality of your everyday life.

## Nutrition Basics

There are six categories of nutrients that your body needs for survival. The four basic nutrients are water, carbohydrates, fats, and proteins. These are called *macronutrients,* because your body requires them daily in large amounts in order to function properly. Water is the most essential macronutrient in maintaining life, even though it contains no energy in the form of calories. Carbohydrates, fats, and proteins supply your body with energy, and serve as the building blocks for growth and repair.

Vitamins and minerals are known as *micronutrients,* because they are needed in relatively small amounts in the body when compared with the macronutrients. Although micronutrients are not considered a source of energy, they are necessary for normal body growth, maintenance, and tissue repair.

It's always better to eat a variety of whole foods so that you get all of the macro- and micronutrients that you need naturally through dietary sources, instead of having to depend on nutrient supplements to make up the difference. Food processing—including refining, enriching, hydrogenating, preserving, and irradiating—can destroy a percentage of the nutrient content of foods. None of these processes enhances the food nutritionally. And, because these processes actually result in considerable loss of nutrients, diets that include too much of these foods supply only the bare minimum of nutrients necessary for survival. So you're better off choosing foods that have undergone minimal—if any—food processing.

It's very important to learn how the food you eat affects your blood glucose levels. You want to recognize how your body responds to different foods, particularly foods containing carbohydrates or proteins. So let's discuss the main nutrients in more detail.

## CARBOHYDRATES

The primary role of carbohydrates is to supply the energy that your body needs to function each day. Most of the glucose in your blood following a meal comes from carbohydrates, which are abundant in plant foods, such as fruits, vegetables, peas, and beans.

Carbohydrates are divided into two groups—simple carbohydrates and complex carbohydrates. Simple carbohydrates, sometimes called simple sugars, consist mainly of single-sugar molecules, and are found mainly in sugar and fruits. Complex carbohydrates are contained in vegetables, as well as whole grains, beans, and legumes. These carbohydrates are made up of long, complex chains of sugars. Therefore, complex carbohydrates take longer to break down than simple sugars. They have to be digested in the stomach and intestines, where they are broken down into single sugar molecules that are more easily absorbed.

Fiber is a complex carbohydrate that your body cannot digest and absorb for energy. However, dietary fiber, which is contained in whole grains, vegetables, fruits, nuts, and seeds, helps the intestines to function efficiently, and aids absorption of sugars into the bloodstream. Fiber-rich diets also promote a feeling of fullness by adding bulk to meals—without adding calories. Some types of dietary fiber can be good for people with diabetes because they can help lower cholesterol levels.

The speed with which glucose gets into the blood does not depend on whether a carbohydrate is simple or complex. What does determine the speed is the amount of carbohydrates you eat at a meal, the way the particular food is prepared, and what combination of foods you eat. For example, the digestion rate is slower for foods that contain fat in addition to carbohydrates. So if you have a food that contains carbohydrates but also contains fat, carbohydrates will be digested more slowly, delaying the change in blood glucose level. Foods that are high in protein can raise blood glucose levels, but not as quickly as foods that contain mostly carbohydrates.

It's normal for carbohydrates to cause blood sugar to rise after a meal. Under normal circumstances, the pancreas secretes enough insulin to allow glucose to enter the body's cells, which in turn reduces blood glucose levels. But the problem with diabetes—as you should know by now—is that insufficient insulin is produced to bring elevated blood glucose levels back down to normal.

## FATS

Lately, there has been a great deal of confusion concerning the place that fats have in the diet. Reports linking high-fat diets to illnesses such as heart disease, certain cancers, and diabetes have driven some people to reduce the fat in their diets to very low levels. However, the fact is that some amount of dietary fat is needed for your body to function properly.

Besides being your body's most concentrated source of energy, with nine calories per gram, fat provides insulation, helps the cells in your body send signals to communicate with other cells, and acts a protective padding for your bones and internal organs. Fats are also components of all cell membranes.

Fat is stored and used as a reserve for energy, so the body always has a backup source of "fuel" when other nutrients, such as carbohydrates, are running low. For example, when insulin levels drop or if carbohydrate intake drops, fat becomes the main source of energy. Unfortunately, the typical American diet includes too much total fat, so that excess fat is stored in the adipose (fat) tissues of the body. A high intake of the wrong kinds of fats can cause blood vessels to become clogged, increasing the risk of heart disease and stroke. And a high-fat diet can lead to obesity, one of the risk factors for type 2 diabetes.

Dietary fat does not directly affect blood sugar levels. It's usually the other components of the meals that cause blood glucose to rise. However, because fats are not digested as quickly as carbohydrates, they can delay the speed with which your blood sugar level rises after you eat a carbohydrate-containing meal. But remember, balance is key! You don't want to increase your fat intake in hopes of keeping your blood sugar level more stable. Indeed, including more fat in your diet will increase your total caloric intake and your blood cholesterol level—as well as your waistline!

Many people who are seeking to reduce their fat intake are including more low-fat and nonfat foods in their diets. While this seems healthful, beware: In many cases, these foods have more sugar than their higher-fat counterparts, so they will actually cause your blood sugar to rise. Low-fat and nonfat foods may contain other ingredients that can affect blood glucose levels, too.

Let's take a closer look at two kinds of fat found in the diet and in the body: triglycerides and cholesterol.

### *Triglycerides*

There are three major types of triglycerides found in the diet and in the body—saturated, polyunsaturated, and monounsaturated.

Saturated fats tend to be solid at room temperature. They are found mainly in animal products, including butter, lard, whole milk, cream, sour cream, cheese, and fatty meats. A diet high in saturated fat can significantly raise blood cholesterol levels, so these fats are considered to be the "bad" fats.

Polyunsaturated fats are generally liquid at room temperature, and are found in corn, soybean, safflower, and sunflower oils. Although these fats have been shown to reduce total blood cholesterol, they may also lower the level of the "good" high-density lipoprotein (HDL) cholesterol (see "Cholesterol," below). Polyunsaturated fats are healthier than saturated fats, but not as healthy as monounsaturated fats, which lower the "bad" low-density lipoprotein (LDL) cholesterol without affecting HDL cholesterol. Olive, peanut, and canola oils have high amounts of monounsaturates, and so do almonds, cashews, peanuts, and pistachios.

### *Cholesterol*

Cholesterol is a fatty substance that has many important functions throughout the body, especially in the creation, maintenance, and repair of cell membranes. It is also used in the formation of hormones such as estrogen, testosterone, progesterone, and cortisol. In the brain and spinal cord, cholesterol serves as part of the insulation that covers nerve cells and keeps nerve signals going to the right locations. Most of the cholesterol in the human body is produced by its own cells, particularly the cells of the liver.

Unfortunately, too many people eat diets overloaded with fat and calories, and as a result get far more of these substances than their bodies can possibly use. Simply put, too much dietary cholesterol in the blood can create some serious problems. And eating too many foods that contain saturated fats compounds this problem, since these types of fats can increase overall blood cholesterol. Excess cholesterol can clog and harden the arteries, increasing the likelihood of heart disease and stroke.

There are two different types of cholesterol—high-density lipoprotein (HDL) cholesterol, and low-density lipoprotein (LDL) cholesterol. HDL cholesterol is often called "good" cholesterol, because it is believed to protect the body by transporting fats, or lipids, through the body. LDL cholesterol, on the other hand, is referred to as "bad" cholesterol, since it tends to deposit fats in the body, increasing the risk of atherosclerosis and other cardiovascular diseases.

## PROTEINS

Protein is necessary for growth and development, and is essential in the repair of cells. All proteins are made up of structural units called amino acids. Of the more than twenty amino acids that have been identified, nine are considered essential amino acids, which cannot be manufactured by the body. Essential amino acids, therefore, must be obtained from dietary sources. Complete proteins are proteins that contain all of the nine essential amino acids in sufficient amounts for adequate growth, development, and cellular repair.

To some extent, amino acids are converted to glucose, and may increase blood glucose levels—but not by much and not quickly. The body tends to spare protein as a source of energy because of the nutrient's importance in growth and development, and its role in the production of hormones, antibodies, enzymes, and body tissues. As such, the body uses mostly carbohydrates and fats for energy, and relies more on protein as the other energy sources are depleted.

Many experts believe that there is more than enough protein in the average American diet, so it's not essential to increase protein intake. In fact, too much protein may be unhealthy, because a high-protein diet tends to put added strain on the kidneys. However, it is important to remember that adequate protein intake is important for a balanced diet. For people with diabetes, protein helps promote a feeling of fullness—an important consideration for anyone following a weight-control program. Also, a meal that contains protein as well as carbohydrates has a gentler effect on blood sugar than an exclusively carbohydrate-rich meal.

Good sources of proteins include milk products, poultry, seafood, beef, pork, eggs, peanut butter, and legumes. Smaller amounts of the nutrient is contained in nuts, vegetables, grains, and bread.

## VITAMINS AND MINERALS

Vitamins are organic (carbon-containing) substances that occur naturally in plants and animals. These nutrients can function as coenzymes in the body—that is, they "help" the enzymes that promote all of the body's biochemical processes, including nerve transmission, muscle contraction, blood formation, protein metabolism, and energy production. Generally speaking, our bodies cannot manufacture vitamins, so we must obtain most of these nutrients from the foods we eat or from vitamin supplements.

Whereas vitamins are organic substances, minerals are inorganic substances, meaning that they are not bound to carbon. Minerals originate in soil and water, and they are absorbed by the plants that are eaten by the animals that make up the human diet. Like vitamins, minerals can function as coenzymes, plus they help build strong bones and teeth and are necessary for the manufacture of hemoglobin, the oxygen-carrying component of blood.

*Antioxidants* are micronutrients that may help protect against a variety of diseases, including heart disease and cancer. Some well known antioxidants include vitamins C and E, and the mineral selenium. These nutrients seem to work by protecting body cells from damage that can be caused by factors such as cigarette smoke, toxic chemicals, and environmental pollution. There is still much to learn about antioxidants and how they function in the body, and scientists are continuing to study the effects of these potentially beneficial nutrients.

A healthy intake of vitamins and minerals is important for everybody, diabetes or no diabetes. If you eat a good variety of nutritious foods—including fresh fruits and vegetables, fiber-rich cereals and grains, and lean cuts of meat—then you're probably getting all of the vitamins and minerals you need to be healthy. There's little scientific evidence to prove that taking in extra amounts of micronutrients, such as through supplementation, can help improve diabetes or maintain blood glucose control. In fact, as important as vitamins and minerals are for health, you need to be prudent about your intake, since some nutrients—such as vitamin A and iron—can actually *cause* health problems when taken in high doses.

If you think that you may not be getting all of the micronutrients you need from dietary sources alone, make an appointment with your dietitian. He or she will be able to educate you about the benefits and possible risks of taking nutritional supplements. Always let your dietitian know what you are already taking; some nutritional supplements can interact with certain drugs and cause potentially dangerous adverse effects. Also, make sure that your supplement plan is customized to fit your age, sex, and medical needs.

If you have high blood pressure, you've probably heard a lot about sodium. Our bodies need some amount of this essential mineral. Sodium helps transport nutrients into cells, so they can be used for energy production, as well as tissue growth and repair. In addition, it helps maintain the volume and balance of all fluids outside the body's cells, such as blood. Unfortunately, too many people include too much sodium in their diets every day.

Some studies have shown that people with diabetes are more sensitive to the blood-pressure-raising effects of sodium than people who do not have diabetes. Because high blood pressure can exacerbate other diabetes-related complications, it's prudent to keep your sodium intake to a minimum. This is not as simple as limiting your intake of table salt, however. There are many foods that naturally contain salt or sodium, and many foods use salt in their preparation, including frankfurters, luncheon meats, and canned vegetables.

Some studies have shown that diets rich in calcium, potassium, and magnesium can help reduce blood pressure. So you can see how a healthy, balanced diet—in combination with exercise and moderate weight loss—can be very beneficial in lowering blood pressure and keeping your cardiovascular system strong.

---

## What About Alcohol?

Alcohol can cause blood sugar levels to drop. Under normal circumstances, when blood glucose levels get too low, the liver converts stored glycogen to glucose and releases it into the bloodstream. However, alcohol interferes with this process, so when your blood sugar level falls, your liver may not be able to release enough glucose to correct the situation. Drinking as little as two to three ounces of alcohol can suppress glucose release from the liver. If your liver is not able to function efficiently, you may become hypoglycemic because of alcohol, although drinking alcohol is a less common cause of hypoglycemia.

Some of the symptoms of hypoglycemia—for example, confusion or slurred speech—may be mistakenly thought to result from drinking alcohol. If this happens, there's a danger that the hypoglycemic episode may progress unrecognized. Hypoglycemia can be a very dangerous condition if left untreated, and can even result in coma or death. (For more information about hypoglycemia, see chapter 10.) Obviously, the most effective way of avoiding this problem is to limit alcohol intake. Additionally, it's a good idea to carry an identification card stating that you have diabetes and that your symptoms may indicate hypoglycemia, which requires immediate medical attention.

So, is it safe to drink alcohol if you have diabetes? The answer is a guarded yes—as long as you are carefully controlling your blood glucose levels. The United States Department of Health and Human Services has stated that one or two drinks a week is not harmful.

Your health-care team can provide you with guidelines that will enable you to include an occasional drink in your meal plan. As a general rule, if you plan to drink alcohol, make sure that you have your drink with a meal, since alcohol intensifies the blood-sugar-lowering effects of insulin. Food provides some of the glucose that your body needs, so the liver will not have to release stored glucose to protect you against hypoglycemia.

---

## A Diet You Can Live With

These days, there are plenty of meal-planning options for people with diabetes. The kinds of foods you will be eating are the same foods recommended for anyone who wants to live a healthy life. You won't have to sustain yourself on special "diet" foods.

For years, the most widely used approach to meal planning for diabetes has been *exchange lists,* which group foods that are similar in nutritional content. These groups are called exchange lists because foods within each list can be exchanged, or substituted, for one another. The six categories included in this approach are: Starches and Grains, Fruits, Milk, Vegetables, Meats and Meat Substitutes, and Fats. Exchange lists offer great flexibility in meal planning because you can select from a variety of foods and still keep the amount of carbohydrates and other nutrients in your meals consistent day to day.

Another meal-planning approach is *carbohydrate counting,* which is based on the rationale that carbohydrates are the main factor affecting blood sugar levels. If you follow this plan, you are allowed a certain number of carbohydrate grams per meal or snack. You keep track of how many carbohydrates you are eating by using a carbohydrate counter book, food labels, or exchange lists. By keeping a count of your carbohydrate intake, you can be sure that you're staying within your carbohydrate budget.

*The First Step in Diabetes Meal Planning* is a joint publication of the American Diabetes Association and the American Dietetic Association. This trifold brochure opens up to display a large poster of the Diabetes Food Guide Pyramid, which is similar to the USDA Food Guide Pyramid. However, starchy vegetables, such as potatoes, corn, and peas, are included in the same group as other high-carbohydrate foods, such as grains, beans, and breads. This makes it easier to plan meals that contain consistent amounts of carbohydrates.

The approaches to meal planning detailed above are just three of many plans that will enable you to meet your nutritional goals. Remember, your approach to meal planning should be tailored to your individual needs based on your average blood sugar level, cholesterol, and triglycerides, as well as your body weight, lifestyle, and food preferences. Your dietitian will work with you to determine which meal-planning approach best fits your needs.

## Diabetes, Pregnancy, and Nutrition

Meal planning for diabetes is a little more complicated if you're pregnant, because you're eating for two. You have to strive to keep your blood sugar stable, as does anyone with diabetes, but at the same time, you need to take in the right amounts of the right nutrients to provide for your health and for the health of your developing baby.

There are no hard-and-fast rules that outline *exactly* what all pregnant women with diabetes should and shouldn't eat. Many factors are taken into consideration in choosing the "best" approach to meal planning. In addition to factoring in your nutritional needs, blood sugar levels, lifestyle, and food preferences, your dietitian and/or nutritionist will need to determine the caloric and nutritional intakes necessary to support the baby's development. (For more on nutritional needs during pregnancy, see chapter 12.)

## Eating Away from Home

Almost anybody with diabetes who is motivated to take charge of his or her health can successfully master meal planning at home. What's more challenging, though, is learning how to eat healthily away from home, such as at a friend's house. Some people with diabetes are afraid that friends will not understand their dietary needs. Others are worried that their friends will have trouble finding foods that are appropriate for a "diabetes-friendly" diet. If you have these or similar concerns, don't despair!

The fact that you have diabetes does not mean you can't enjoy dinner with your friends. You just have to plan for these special occasions. For instance, if you know *where* you're going to eat, you can plan *what* you're going to eat. But even if you're not certain about what's going to be available, you can still make some accommodations by adjusting the rest of your treatment program. You might compensate by reducing the amount that you eat of other types of foods. Your physician, dietitian, or diabetes educator can give you specific tips and guidelines to help you enjoy these special events.

Plenty of people out there equate eating out with splurging. However, since restaurant meals have become a regular part of the American lifestyle, this isn't really a healthful practice for anyone. Think about how many times you eat restaurant meals—including fast food—each week. Which restaurants do you choose? What foods do you order? You may well be sabotaging your own efforts to stick to a healthy meal plan.

Lots of people who eat restaurant meals have concerns about their health and need to ask questions about what's on the menu, and a growing number of establishments are keeping up with consumer demand for healthy foods. But even if a restaurant doesn't have any special low-fat or healthy items, there are many strategies you can use to make sure you get what you want when you dine out.

- If you're going to a restaurant you've never tried before, call ahead to find out about menu options and whether foods are appropriate for your meal plan.
- Don't be afraid to ask about ingredients and to get foods made to order. For example, request to have your dish prepared without butter or salt, or that sauces, dressings, and margarine or butter are served on the side or left off altogether.
- Steer clear of high-fat foods and high-fat preparation methods. Avoid items that are served in butter, cream, or cheese sauce, marinated in oil, or fried. And don't succumb to the temptation of foods that are battered or breaded, or are described as flaky, crispy, or creamy—these are often loaded with fat because of the way they're prepared.
- Look for menu items that are steamed, broiled, blackened, grilled, roasted, stir-fried, stewed, braised, or in their own juices.
- If you tend to overeat at restaurants, set goals for yourself—and stick to them! Stop eating when you are comfortably full. Most restaurants have take-home containers available, so your left-overs needn't go to waste.

It's a good idea to jot down a summary of your diet plan on a card that you can take with you wherever you go. This way, it's easy to make sure that what you'd like to order can be included in your meal plan—just refer to the card. If you know, for example, that the portion you have been served is too large, cut that part of the meal that is excessive and move it to another plate before you even begin eating.

No matter how committed you are to following your meal plan, there will be times when you decide to be a little indulgent. For example, if you're going to a party or another special event, and you know you'll be eating more than usual, plan to compensate. At an other times, you may find yourself facing some circumstances you just can't control—situations where sticking to your healthy eating plan is just impossible. For instance, if you will be having your meal later than ususal, have a small snack that contains starch or sugar to tide you over until it's time to eat. This will prevent hypoglycemia and take the edge off your hunger so you'll have more control when ordering. Finally, always carry snacks with you—you never know when you may get stuck in traffic or be delayed for other reasons.

## A Culinary Conclusion

So what's the moral? By understanding basics about nutrition and meal plans, not only will you eat a well-balanced healthy diet but you'll also help to keep your blood sugar in control. Eat healthily, eat properly, eat in moderation, and enjoy!

# CHAPTER NINE

# Following Your Exercise Program

Regular exercise is good for everyone. It helps us look and feel better about ourselves, and it increases cardiorespiratory fitness, aids in weight control, and improves muscle tone. For people with diabetes, exercise is especially important because it can help improve blood glucose control, which reduces the risk of diabetes-related complications.

Maybe you've been motivated to start exercising, only to find that your motivation quickly dissipated. Or maybe you've put off starting a workout program altogether. It's easy to find excuses not to exercise. How many times have you talked yourself out of exercising by falling back on the old standbys "I'm too tired" or "I don't have time today" or even "It probably won't work, anyway"? That's not uncommon. However, it's important to realize that regular physical activity is an integral part of your treatment program, and it's an aspect that you can't afford to neglect—for you health's sake. Whether you've tried an exercise program and failed to stick with it, or this is your first foray into the fitness world, this chapter will show you that there's no excuse not to exercise.

## Benefits of Exercise

For people with diabetes, one of the most important benefits of regular physical activity is improved blood sugar control. Exercise makes your muscles work harder, so your body uses more "fuel" in the form of sugar. This reduces the amount of sugar in your bloodstream. Plus, exercise increases the body cells' sensitivity to insulin. As a result, less insulin is needed to help glucose move from the blood into the cells.

Exercise can lower "bad" LDL cholesterol and triglyceride levels, and raise "good" HDL cholesterol, which eliminates fatty deposits from the arteries. Regular physical activity can also help control high blood pressure and decrease clotting in the blood. And exercise strengthens the heart muscle. All of these benefits reduce the risk of cardiovascular disease. This is good news for all of us, of course, but it's especially helpful to people with diabetes, who have an increased risk of heart attack and stroke.

If weight loss is one of your goals, regular exercise—in combination with a healthful eating plan—will enable you to reach and maintain your ideal weight. Because you burn extra calories and fat when you exercise, your body loses fat and increases in muscle mass. Exercise will also raise your metabolism, so your body will burn more calories, even when you're not working out.

Exercise is as important for your state of mind as it is for your body. Sure, you'll feel better physically—and you'll like what you see, too! Your self-esteem is sure to get a boost when you start to notice the results of your commitment to exercise. Working out can help relieve stress and tension, and ease feelings of depression, anger, fear, and frustration. Exercise can also help you to enjoy deep sleep, so you'll be able to face each day fully rested.

When you consider all of the physical and psychological benefits of exercise, it's clear that the right workout program can improve the quality of your life.

## SPECIFICS FOR TYPE 1 DIABETES

If you have type 1 diabetes, exercise alone will not improve blood glucose control. That doesn't mean that there's no good reason to start an exercise program, however. Quite the contrary! Regular physical activity will help keep your weight under control, and it will keep your heart beating strong and healthy, reducing your risk of developing long-term diabetes-related complications such as cardiovascular disease. Exercise may even enable you to lower your regular dose of insulin. (But remember that you shouldn't make *any* adjustments in your medications without the advice and supervision of your health-care practitioner!)

Hypoglycemia is a very real risk for active people with type 1 diabetes. Adding exercise to your diabetes care plan will require the careful balance of food, insulin, and physical activity, so it's especially important to work with your health-care team when you plan a workout program. Your doctor or diabetes educator can give you vital information on how to decrease your insulin or increase your calories to compensate for the blood-glucose-lowering effects of exercise. You will also need to discuss when you should exercise in relation to when you eat.

## SPECIFICS FOR TYPE 2 DIABETES

Weight control is a primary goal for the majority of people with type 2 diabetes. As any member of your treatment team can tell you, starting a carefully planned program of diet and exercise—and sticking with it!—is the best way to reach and maintain your ideal weight. And, for many people with type 2 diabetes, making the commitment to a more healthful lifestyle means better blood glucose control—without the need for insulin or oral diabetes medication. Good control reduces your risk of developing short- and long-term complications of diabetes.

If you have type 2 diabetes and you use insulin or oral diabetes medications, be aware that you'll need to take some precautions when you exercise, to minimize your risk of hypoglycemia. Talk to your doctor or diabetes educator to find out the best way to balance your food, medication, and exercise to keep your blood sugar from dropping too low.

## Types of Exercise

Exercise can be divided into two categories—*aerobic* and *anaerobic.* Aerobic exercises are vigorous exercises that require the body to use increased amounts of oxygen, which makes your heart and lungs work harder and keeps your cardiovascular system in peak operating condition. Fast walking, running, swimming, dancing, step aerobics, and bicycling are examples of aerobic exercise. When you engage in these types of activities, your muscles become more attuned to burning fat, and they will increase their fat-burning activity at rest.

Anaerobic exercise requires shorter bursts of activity that can build strength, increase flexibility, and improve muscle tone and coordination. One good example of anaerobic activity is strength training, which makes the muscles work against resistance. Strength training—for example, weight lifting or push-ups—is the most effective type of exercise you can do to build and maintain muscle mass.

Because weight control is an important goal for a great many people with diabetes, aerobic exercise is generally considered to be more beneficial. Plus, aerobic activities lower blood glucose and improve cardiovascular function. As you've already learned, all of these benefits are essential to the continued health of people with diabetes.

## Getting Started

Before you begin any exercise program, you should schedule a complete physical to make sure that exercising is safe for you. Your physician or exercise specialist can help you develop an appropriate exercise regimen based on the type and severity of your diabetes, any other medical conditions you may have, the medications you're taking (if any), whether you're overweight, the types of activities you enjoy, and your overall physical condition.

If you have a diabetes-related complication, you can still choose an exercise program, but you need to make sure that the activity you choose is appropriate—that is, that your exercise regimen will not contribute to further harm. It's very important that you're clear on which activities are safe for you, so you must work closely with your health-care team to plan a program that will provide maximum benefits with little or no risk.

For your exercise program to be successful, you'll need to start slowly and gradully build up your endurance and intensity over several weeks or months. The idea is to give your body time to become accustomed to physical activity so that you won't overexert yourself. If you try to do too much too fast, you run a greater risk of injury. Set *realistic* goals for yourself so that you'll stay motivated. If you expect to see fantastic results after only a short period of time, you may feel frustrated and be less tempted to stick to your program.

## Exercising Caution

You should always warm up before beginning any type of exercise. A good warm-up should include a variety of stretches and a few minutes of gradually increasing, low-intensity activity. Stretching increases blood flow to the muscles and will increase the temperature of the tendons the muscles are attached to, making it less likely the muscles will be pulled to the point of injury during exercise. Then you'll be ready to participate in twenty to thirty minutes or more of aerobic activity to get your heart pumping and your blood flowing.

Exercise at a rate at which you can comfortably carry on a conversation. If you feel weak, become short of breath, or have any pain, stop immediately. When you have finished your exercise routine, take another five to ten minutes for a cool-down period. Light stretching during this time will reduce soreness and increase flexibility.

In addition to these precautions, there are some other measures you should take that will ensure your safety when you exercise.

## MONITOR YOUR BLOOD GLUCOSE

Starting an exercise program means that you will have to monitor your blood glucose more frequently—before and after your workout, and sometimes during exercise, if it's of long duration. This is very important, because you want to get an idea of how exercise affects your blood sugar level.

Physical activity usually causes blood glucose levels to drop, so if your blood sugar is already low you may want to have a snack before your workout; otherwise, you may be putting yourself at risk for a hypoglycemic episode. Furthermore, you should not exercise if your blood sugar is above 240 mg/dl and you have ketones in your urine. If your blood sugar is this high, exercise can cause your blood sugar and ketones to rise even higher.

Always take a snack along when you exercise, in case you feel a hypoglycemic episode coming on. Glucose tablets, hard candies, and raisins are easy to carry and should work well to raise your blood sugar if it drops too low. If you experience any symptoms that may indicate low blood sugar during exercise, stop immediately. As soon as possible, test your blood sugar, and eat one of your fast-acting sugar snacks if necessary.

The blood glucose-lowering effects of exercise may last for several hours after your workout, because your muscles take up glucose from the blood to replenish the glucose that your body used during exercise. For this reason, you need to be on the alert for signs of hypoglycemia even after you've finished exercising for the day.

## DRINK PLENTY OF WATER

Water is involved in almost every function of the body. When you exercise, your body loses water through sweating and evaporation. Sweat is your body's coolant, and is therefore an essential mechanism for regulating body temperature. As such, replacing water that is continuously lost through sweating is very important.

Dehydration can put you at risk of overheating, especially if you're exercising in hot weather. Although it may be impossible to offset all the water lost through sweating, even partial replacement can minimize the risk of overheating. To be safe, make sure you're well hydrated before you exercise. If you will be exercising for a long duration, make sure you have water with you so you can replenish lost fluids during your workout. And don't wait until you're thirsty to take a drink—thirst is often a sign that you're already dehydrated.

## LISTEN TO YOUR BODY

If you're just starting an exercise program, you should expect to feel some minor discomfort from exercising. This is only natural, since your body is not used to regular physical activity. Despite the fact that some amount of muscle soreness is a normal result of exercise, you shouldn't ignore this discomfort. Listen to your body. If the pain is moderate or severe, or if your aches and pains aren't going away, your body's telling you that you're overdoing it, so you should take a day or two off. Also, take a break from your exercise program if you have an injury, such as a sprain or muscle strain. You need to give your body time to heal. And skip your workout if you're feeling ill, because you don't want to make the situation worse. But make sure your "vacation" is a short one—it's easy to get out of the exercise habit!

## CARRY IDENTIFICATION

Always carry identification and diabetes information with you when you exercise. This way, you'll be more likely to receive proper assistance if you are in a situation in which you can't help yourself. Include your name, address, phone number, physician's name and phone number, and type and dose of insulin or other diabetes medications.

## SELECT THE RIGHT FOOTWEAR

Invest in good gear for your feet. If your exercise program involves activities that are stressful to your feet, you have to protect them. Select comfortable, high-quality shoes fitted by a competent salesperson. Also, check your feet before and after exercise to be sure that you don't have blisters, cuts, or any developing problems.

## Staying with the Program

Despite all of the benefits of exercise, a lot of people have trouble sticking with their workout programs. Some complain that exercise is boring; others focus on the things they'd rather be doing; still others say there just isn't enough time in each day to work out. But it's important to realize that, when it comes to your health, there's no room for excuses. If you want to take control of your diabetes and be as healthy as you can be, then you need to start a program of regular exercise.

Try some of the following tips, and you may find that it's not so difficult to make exercise a regular part of your life.

- Set up a workout schedule and stick with it. Remind yourself that exercise is a priority and is just as important as any other activity or appointment you may have during the day.
- Add variety to your exercise program. Exercise should be fun. Choose activities that you enjoy, and alternate exercises daily. This will keep you from getting bored with your exercise program, and ensure that you don't overwork a particular part of your body.
- Set specific, short-term goals to keep yourself motivated, and stay focused on achieving these goals. Long-term goals are good, too, but if they seem too distant and unachievable, you might get discouraged when you don't see immediate progress.
- Reward yourself for sticking with your exercise program. Sometimes we all need artificial incentives to do things that we may not otherwise want to do. Every so often, buy yourself a book or CD that you've had your eye on.
- Keep track of your progress. Write down what kind of exercise you did, at what intensity, and for how long. Keeping an exercise journal will enable you to see the progress you've made, and this will help you stay motivated.

- Exercise with a buddy. Make a commitment with each other to stick with the exercise program. Also, a training partner who is aware of your diabetes can help ensure your safety when you work out. Your friend can help you (or get help for you) should you be unable to help yourself.

## A Final Exercise

Because every person is different, there is no one set of exercises that can be recommended for everyone. But everybody is capable of doing some exercises, and everybody can benefit from them. Just don't jump in feet-first! Use your head. Work with your physician or exercise therapist to choose an exercise regimen that will help you achieve your fitness goals. Then start slowly, build up your stamina, and enjoy your improved health!

## CHAPTER TEN

# Preventing Short-Term Complications

The most common short-term complications of diabetes are high blood sugar (hyperglycemia) and low blood sugar (hypoglycemia). These are potentially life-threatening problems. While many people can feel a hyperglycemic or hypoglycemic episode coming on, some people have high or low blood sugar levels without experiencing any warning symptoms. That's why it's so important to check your blood sugar regularly. This chapter discusses the causes, symptoms, and treatment of high and low blood sugar.

## What Is Hyperglycemia?

If your blood glucose level rises above 250 mg/dl, or is at or above 180 mg/dl at the same time of day for three days in a row, you are considered to have hyperglycemia, or high blood sugar. Hyperglycemia may come on suddenly, or its onset may be more gradual—but either way, high blood sugar is not to be taken lightly. In the short-term, elevated blood sugar levels may cause diabetic ketoacidosis, generally in people with type 1 diabetes, or a condition known as hyperglycemic hyperosmolar syndrome (HHS), which occurs in people with type 2 diabetes. Prolonged hyperglycemia, lasting over the course of several years, can lead to diabetic complications such as damage to blood vessels and nerves throughout the body. You'll learn more about the long-term complications of diabetes in chapter 11. For now, we're going to focus on the more immediate consequences of high blood sugar.

## CAUSES OF HYPERGLYCEMIA

Hyperglycemia is not always preventable, even for people who are very vigilant about keeping their blood sugar levels under control. However, it's important to be aware of the circumstances that may lead to hyperglycemia so that you can take measures to reduce its occurrence. The causes of hyperglycemia include:

- Eating the wrong foods.
- Eating too much of the right foods.
- Lack of exercise.
- Psychological or emotional stress.
- Physical stress, such as illness or injury.
- Taking too much or too little medication.

## SYMPTOMS OF HYPERGLYCEMIA

Although some people do not notice any symptoms of hyperglycemia, others do experience some of the same symptoms that led to their initial diagnosis of diabetes. Usually, the warning signs of a hyperglycemic episode include one or more of the following symptoms:

- Frequent urination.
- Excessive thirst.
- Frequent or excessive hunger.
- Blurred vision.
- Fatigue.
- Confused thinking.

If you develop any of the symptoms listed on page 111, you should take immediate actions to bring your blood sugar level under control. If you ignore these symptoms, you may very well have to deal with a more severe complication.

## WHAT TO DO ABOUT HYPERGLYCEMIA

The best thing you can do when your blood glucose level begins to rise is to check you blood sugar more frequently. If you find that it's consistently over 140 or 150 mg/dl or if it's over 240 mg/dl twice in a row, call your doctor and get instructions on how to handle the problem. Make sure that you are taking your medication at the right times and in the right amounts, and be very careful to follow your diet plan.

If your blood sugar is over 240 mg/dl, check for ketones in your urine. Contact your physician immediately if ketones are present in your urine, as this may indicate that you are developing diabetic ketoacidosis, a serious complication of diabetes that is discussed in the next section. Do not exercise if your blood sugar is this high, because exercise can cause an increase in both blood glucose and ketone levels.

## PROBLEMS ASSOCIATED WITH HYPERGLYCEMIA

If you are unable to keep your blood sugar level controlled—even despite your best efforts—you should be aware of the acute complications that may develop. It's important to realize that early intervention is the key to preventing these conditions, which include diabetic ketoacidosis and hyperglycemic hyperosmolar syndrome. And it's equally essential to be able to recognize the symptoms of these complications so that you can take the appropriate measures to handle any situation. Let's start by taking a closer look at diabetic ketoacidosis.

### *Diabetic Ketoacidosis*

Diabetic ketoacidosis typically occurs only in people with type 1 diabetes who have high, uncontrolled blood sugar levels. DKA is a condition in which the blood becomes acidic due to high levels of ketones in the bloodstream. Without treatment, DKA may progress to coma in a matter of hours.

As you've already learned, insulin is necessary for the body's cells to burn sugar. Without insulin, the cells are not able to burn sugar for energy and the body looks to fat as another source of energy. When insulin is not available to help cells absorb glucose, the body has to burn fat as an alternate energy source. The body always burns some fat as fuel, even in people who don't have diabetes. Therefore, there is always a certain level of ketones in the bloodstream. However, the increased breakdown of fat causes ketones to accumulate in the bloodstream. Eventually, ketones begin to spill over into the urine as more and more fat is burned as fuel.

The real danger occurs when ketones build up in the body faster than they can be eliminated through the urine. Because of the acidic products contained in the ketones, higher levels of ketones can cause the entire body to become too acidic. This is what we know as DKA. This condition requires *immediate* treatment.

Diabetic ketoacidosis suggests the presence of far too little insulin in the blood. If you take insulin at the proper times and in the right dosages, then the development of DKA may suggest that your body needs more insulin than you're currently taking. DKA may also develop during periods of illness or stress.

***Symptoms of DKA.*** Diabetic ketoacidosis can be prevented if you're aware of the warning signs of hyperglycemia, and you take measures to bring your blood glucose level back down to your target range. Of course, the most significant sign that you may be headed for trouble is a blood glucose level above 240 mg/dl. If you monitor your blood sugar at the same times each and every day, you won't miss this signal. Also, take note of any possible symptoms of hyperglycemia that you might be experiencing (see page 111). If you're observant, you'll detect hyperglycemia before it can cause further problems.

Should you fail to recognize that your blood sugar is out of control, you may begin to experience symptoms of DKA, including:

- Loss of appetite.
- Nausea or vomiting.
- Pain and cramping in the stomach.
- A flushed appearance to the skin.
- Tiredness and weakness.
- Dehydration.
- Deep, rapid breathing.
- A fruity smell on your breath.

***What to Do About DKA.*** Proper medical attention is essential in cases of DKA. Whether or not you have any of the above symptoms, call your doctor without delay if you have blood glucose results over 240 mg/dl and ketones in your urine. *Do not* ignore the warning signs of DKA, as this is a potentially deadly condition. Drink plenty of water (or fluid that doesn't contain sugar) to prevent dehydration, and avoid exercise, which can cause your blood glucose and ketone levels to rise even higher.

DKA often requires immediate medical attention in the hospital. The primary components of treatment are to provide additional insulin, increase levels of fluids, and make sure that electrolytes—especially potassium—do not fall too low.

### *Hyperglycemic Hyperosmolar Syndrome*

Hyperglycemic hyperosmolar syndrome is seen most often in people with type 2 diabetes. For the most part, it occurs in people who have not been taking proper care of their diabetes. HHS may also be caused by alcohol use, inadequate fluid intake, loss of large amounts of fluid, untreated infections, and other physical stressors. Many cases occur in people who don't even know they have diabetes.

In HHS, blood sugar rises so high that the blood actually becomes thicker. Extreme high levels of glucose in the blood, in combination with loss of fluids, can lead to this condition. As blood glucose levels increase, the output of urine increases, and dehydration results. Extreme dehydration may lead to confusion or to mental changes that are similar to those experienced by stroke victims. This, in turn, can make the person with HHS unable to help him or herself, and the condition worsens.

***Symptoms of HHS.*** The symptoms of HHS are, for the most part, similar to the symptoms of DKA; however, if ketones are present, there are only small amounts. Of course, abnormally high blood glucose is the first sign. Other indicators of HHS include:

- Extreme thirst
- Dry mouth
- Confusion
- Tiredness or weakness
- Warm, dry skin with no sweating

If your blood glucose level exceeds 350 mg/dl contact your doctor immediately. He or she will explain the steps you should take to bring your blood sugar back down to within your target range. If your blood glucose level rises over 500 mg/dl, have someone take you to the hospital immediately.

***What to Do About HHS.*** Just like DKA, hyperglycemic hyperosmolar syndrome can be prevented. The surest way to avoid developing this condition is to monitor your blood glucose regularly and frequently. Remember, your goal is to keep your blood sugar level within your target range. If you realize that your blood glucose is abnormally high, you can take measures to bring the level back down before more serious complications develop. It's especially important to monitor blood glucose frequently during illness, since this kind of physical stress can cause blood glucose levels to become elevated. Make sure you drink plenty of water (or fluids that don't contain sugar), and avoid alcohol and caffeine.

HHS is a medical emergency. The condition can be fatal if it's not treated promptly in the hospital, so *do not* ignore the symptoms if they should arise. Patients are given fluids for rehydration and insulin to get their blood glucose levels down, and their electrolytes are monitored.

# What Is Hypoglycemia?

Hypoglycemia, or low blood sugar, is the most common complication of diabetes treatment with oral medications or insulin. The symptoms usually occur when blood sugar levels are below 70 mg/dl. This complication is seen more often in people with type 1 diabetes—estimates are that people with type 1 diabetes may have one or two hypoglycemic episodes each week. However, people with type 2 diabetes may develop this condition, as well.

Hypoglycemia comes on suddenly and progresses through three stages: mild, moderate, and severe. In its most severe form, low blood sugar is very dangerous, and can cause disorientation, unconsciousness, seizures, and even coma. This is why it's so important to treat this complication immediately.

## CAUSES OF HYPOGLYCEMIA

Hypoglycemia is caused by one or a combination of a number of factors, including taking too high a dose of insulin or oral diabetes medications; skipping meals or eating too little food; and exercising strenuously or doing more physical activity than usual. Drinking alcohol or taking certain prescription and over-the-counter drugs can also cause your blood sugar level to drop dangerously low. Additionally, people that have problems with food absorption are more likely to experience hypoglycemia, because their bodies may not absorb enough glucose from food.

As discussed in chapter 6, people who follow a program of intensive insulin therapy have an increased chance of developing hypoglycemia. Remember, the goal of tight control is to maintain blood sugar levels as near normal as possible by monitoring blood glucose several times a day, and making adjustments in insulin based on food choices, exercise, and glucose test results. Because overall blood glucose levels are kept within a lower range, it's easier for these levels to slip even lower.

Keeping blood sugar under control without allowing the level to drop too low can be challenging, since the amount of insulin your body needs is variable. Your choice of food and how much you eat, the timing of your insulin or other medication, your emotions, when and how much you exercise, the amount of stress you're under, and the overall state of your health all affect your blood glucose level and, as such, how much insulin you need to keep the level within your target range. No matter how hard you try, you can't keep tight control over every one of these factors—it's just not possible for anyone. Consequently, it's impossible to eliminate all hypoglycemic episodes.

Virtually anyone who is taking insulin or pills to control diabetes has an increased risk of hypoglycemia. Anybody who is at risk should know how to recognize the symptoms of hypoglycemia, in order to treat the problem before it becomes too serious.

## SYMPTOMS OF HYPOGLYCEMIA

If your blood sugar level falls too low, you may begin to experience some physical, mental, or emotional symptoms. However, it is possible to have hypoglycemia without feeling or showing any symptoms, so it's very important to check your blood sugar regularly, according to the advice of your diabetes treatment team. Usually, the warning signs of a hypoglycemic episode include one or more of the following symptoms:

- Shakiness.
- Sweating.
- Pounding or rapid heartbeat.
- Blurry vision.
- Headache.
- Dizziness or light-headedness.
- Poor coordination.
- Extreme hunger.
- Severe fatigue.
- Confusion.
- Difficulty concentrating.
- Slurred or slowed speech.
- Irritability.

Hypoglycemia can impair your ability to carry out normal activities. Driving a car, operating machinery, and even cooking can be dangerous if your blood sugar level drops below a normal range. Confusion and an inability to think clearly can also interfere with your ability to recognize that you're experiencing hypoglycemic symptoms, and to make sure the condition is treated properly. Family members, friends, or coworkers may recognize the mental and emotional signs of hypoglycemia even before you do. They may notice that you are confused or disoriented, or that you are unusually "emotional" or irritable.

Symptoms of mild hypoglycemia are primarily physical—trembling, sweatiness, headache, and so forth. You may notice that you are not thinking quite as clearly as you usually do, or that your behavior is just a little different. Because these changes are usually subtle, those around you may not be aware that anything is unusual.

Moderate hypoglycemia can cause you to act confused or to behave inappropriately. Although this is more serious than mild hypoglycemia, it's not so severe that you're not able to take care of yourself. Should you experience severe hypoglycemia, you will need help from others, since you may be too confused and disoriented to act on your own behalf. There's also the possibility that you may lose consciousness. Your family, friends, and coworkers should know how to help you in case of emergency. (See "Administering Glucagon" on page 122.)

## WHAT TO DO ABOUT HYPOGLYCEMIA

Obviously, prevention is the key to dealing with hypoglycemia. To keep your blood sugar from falling too low, eat your meals at around the same times each day—*never* skip meals. Recognize that hunger may be a sign your blood sugar level is too low, and that you need to take steps to bring it back up to within a normal range. Also, make sure you take your medication as directed, in the correct dosage and at the proper times. And be vigilant about monitoring your blood sugar levels. This way, you'll be able to detect low blood sugar, even if you aren't experiencing any overt symptoms.

If you feel that you are developing hypoglycemia, check your blood sugar if you have a monitor available. If for some reason you can't check your blood sugar, go ahead and treat yourself as if you do have low blood sugar. You don't want the condition to progress—especially to the level at which you would be unable to take care of yourself.

Be careful about the possibility of developing hypoglycemia during or after exercise, since physical activity lowers blood glucose levels. Don't work out so hard that you risk reducing your blood sugar to a dangerous range, especially if you're exercising by yourself. If you know that your workout is going to be rigorous enough to burn a lot of calories, make sure that you have a snack beforehand. Because research suggests that hypoglycemia is more likely to occur four to ten hours after exercise than during or shortly after exercise, you may want to monitor your blood sugar levels to look for patterns as to how exercise affects your body. Should you experience any symptoms of low blood sugar during your workout, stop exercising immediately. Don't try to do "just a little bit more."

Cutting back on your alcohol consumption will also help reduce your risk of low blood sugar. Under normal circumstances, when blood glucose levels get too low, the liver converts stored glycogen to glucose and releases it into the bloodstream. However, alcohol interferes with this process, so when your blood sugar level falls, your liver may not be able to release enough glucose to correct the situation.

Because it's not possible to completely eliminate the chance of experiencing hypoglycemia, always be prepared to treat this potentially dangerous complication. You should carry with you—or have access to—a fast-acting source of sugar that will quickly bring your blood glucose level up to a safe range. If you recognize the symptoms of hypoglycemia, quickly eat or drink something containing 10 to 15 grams of simple carbohydrate. Choose one of the following:

- One-half cup of regular (not sugar-free) soft drink.
- One-half cup of orange juice or apple juice.
- Five to seven Life Savers or other sugar candies.
- Ten gumdrops.
- Six jelly beans.
- Two tablespoons (or a small box) of raisins.

- Two teaspoons of honey.
- One cup of skim or 1-percent milk.
- One tablespoon (3 packets) of granulated sugar or six half-inch sugar cubes.
- Three to four glucose tablets.

After you consume your ten to fifteen grams of fast-acting sugars, rest for about fifteen minutes, and then check your blood sugar level again. If low blood sugar is not corrected after this time, repeat the treatment described above. After you have brought your blood sugar level up to normal, you may want to have a snack if it's still a while before your next meal.

Even though it's so important to treat hypoglycemia immediately, you should avoid overtreating the condition. Remember, your goal is to bring your blood sugar back up to a normal range, not to cause it to shoot up above normal levels. So don't go overboard on sweet foods—especially if you're trying to lose weight!

Sometimes, people are so afraid of low blood sugar that they will purposely keep their blood sugar levels higher than normal in order to avoid a possible hypoglycemic episode. This is not a good idea, because high blood sugar comes with its own special set of problems, including an increased risk of long-term complications.

## HYPOGLYCEMIA UNAWARENESS

The ability to recognize the early warning signs of hypoglycemia varies from person to person. Some people have a more difficult time recognizing the symptoms and understanding that a hypoglycemic episode is going to occur. *Hypoglycemia unawareness* develops in some people with diabetes. As the name implies, people with this problem fail to detect any symptoms of low blood sugar. The danger is that if the early warning signs of hypoglycemia go unrecognized, a more severe hypoglycemic episode may result.

Hypoglycemia unawareness is most often a problem for people who have had diabetes for a number of years—usually fifteen to twenty years or more. In these people, hypoglycemia seems to occur with very little warning, because they can no longer recognize many of the symptoms that are indicative of the early stages of hypoglycemia. Why does this happen? Many experts believe that hypoglycemia unawareness is usually the result of neuropathy, or nerve damage—a long-term complication of diabetes. As a result of this damage, adrenaline is not released as it normally would be, and the adrenaline-related symptoms of low blood sugar, such as rapid heartbeat, trembling, or sweatiness, don't become apparent. Instead, people with this problem only experience the mental symptoms of hypoglycemia, such as confusion. At this stage, hypoglycemia may have already progressed to a moderate or severe state.

It's especially important to test your blood sugar several times a day if you are one of the people who cannot recognize the early stages of hypoglycemia. This way, even if you're not aware of the symptoms, the numbers will indicate whether or not your blood sugar level is too low.

Make sure to check your blood sugar before you drive, just to be certain that your level is not dipping too low; if you have a hypoglycemic episode when you're behind the wheel of a car, you run the risk of getting into an accident and hurting yourself or someone else. If you're going to be driving a long distance, make sure you eat small snacks to keep your blood sugar within a normal range. It's also a good idea to place a card on the windshield or dashboard of your car that explains your condition and the treatment necessary. The card should include your doctor's name and phone number.

Because you may experience low blood sugar during sleep, you are advised to check your blood glucose at night before you go to bed. Hypoglycemia during sleep is potentially very dangerous, because you will not be awake and able to take steps to treat the problem. If your blood glucose level at bedtime is below 120 mg/dl, especially if you are active during the day, you may want to have a snack before you go to bed.

Remember, let your family, friends, and coworkers know about the possibility that you will experience hypoglycemia, and tell them about the symptoms that may occur if you do develop this complication.

## Administering Glucagon

When your blood sugar dips below a set point, your pancreas responds by secreting the hormone glucagon. Glucagon inhibits insulin release and causes liver cells to break down stored glycogen into glucose, which is released into the bloodstream. Glucagon works unless the person has no glucose stored in the liver.

If you develop hypoglycemia and can't swallow, or if you become unconscious, an injection of glucagon can quickly raise your blood sugar. Glucagon comes premeasured in a kit, so it is safe to use without the danger of overdosing, and it can last for several years when stored in the refrigerator. Make sure that you have someone with you as often as possible who knows what to do with the glucagon if it becomes necessary. Family members, friends, and coworkers should learn how to give you a glucagon injection in case of an emergency. However, make sure that these individuals know to call for emergency help at once if any problems arise. Also make sure they know that if you are nonresponsive for fifteen to thirty minutes, they should call for emergency assistance.

Responses to glucagon usually occur within five to twenty minutes. Be aware that you may experience an upset stomach after receiving glucagon. You may even vomit. Because of this, your head should be elevated above body level, and you should have crackers or soda to consume as soon as you are alert and able to swallow. Then, as soon as you're able to eat something more substantial than crackers or soda, you should have a substantial snack. In addition, make sure you let your doctor know that you had a severe enough hypoglycemia attack to require a glucagon injection.

## Always Be Prepared

When you have diabetes, it's vital that you be aware of the effects it can have on your body, particularly in terms of your blood glucose levels. Knowing the warning signs that your blood glucose is rising or falling to dangerous levels may save your life. Remember to check your blood glucose at regular intervals so you can catch the first sign of high or low levels. This way you'll be aware of the situation, even if you aren't experiencing any warning symptoms. And always test more frequently if you find that your blood glucose is getting out of control.

## CHAPTER ELEVEN

# Preventing or Controlling Long-Term Complications

The possibility of developing long-term complications is one of the most frightening aspects of diabetes. Prolonged periods of high blood sugar increase the risk of complications in people with diabetes. Common ailments include cardiovascular disease, (such as hypertension and atherosclerosis), eye disorders, kidney disease, nerve disorders, and foot and lower leg problems. Most of these conditions result from years of chronic high blood sugar levels.

The more you know about the complications of diabetes, the better prepared you'll be to prevent them. When you make the commitment to take good care of yourself, you'll be taking a big step toward a better quality of life in the future. Of course, there are some factors—including your age, race, and genetic background—that can put you at greater risk of developing complications, despite your best efforts at managing your diabetes. But this doesn't mean you should give up on your self-management program. Even if you are unable to prevent certain complications, there are certainly measures you can take to minimize their effects, so you should be prepared to deal with any problems that may develop.

# Cardiovascular Disease

People with diabetes are two to four times more likely to develop heart disease than people who do not have diabetes, and five times more likely to have a stroke. Statistics show that more than half the deaths in older people with diabetes are due to cardiovascular disease.

Most cardiovascular complications occur when blood vessels become too narrow or are clogged, or the blood itself becomes too thick. This reduces or even blocks blood flow to the heart, brain, and other important organs and tissues. When blood flow to the heart is slowed for a period of time, one result is a kind of chest pain called *angina.* Although angina is not a disease, it is a warning signal that something is reducing the flow of blood to the heart.

Symptoms that may indicate heart disease include a feeling of pressure in the chest, especially during or after exercise; severe chest pain that starts in the chest and radiates to the shoulders, neck, arms, or hands, fainting spells, difficulty breathing, sweating, nausea with chest discomfort, light-headedness, and irregular heartbeat.

In diagnosing possible cardiovascular disease, doctors may order an electrocardiogram (EKG)—a test that measures the heart's electrical patterns—to determine whether there is any damage to your heart. In addition, doctors may also want you to have an exercise tolerance test—also called a stress test—which measures the effectiveness of your heart muscle when you are under the stress of exercising. It usually involves walking on a treadmill while being monitored by a continuous EKG.

Let's discuss two types of cardiovascular complications that can result from diabetes: hypertension and atherosclerosis.

## HYPERTENSION

Blood pressure, the force exerted by the blood against arterial walls, is what keeps blood circulating. If the pressure is too high, it places a strain on the arteries that can lead to serious problems throughout the body. Of all the risk factors for cardiovascular disease, hypertension (high blood pressure) is one of the greatest.

High blood pressure is very common among people with diabetes. In many cases, the condition does not produce outward symptoms, so many people are not even aware that they have it. Therefore, hypertension may go undiscovered until detected during a routine physical or an examination for another heart problem. It's estimated that 60 percent of people with type 2 diabetes may have high blood pressure. The percentage for people with type 1 diabetes is lower than this; however, in people with type 1 diabetes, hypertension may be a sign of kidney disease.

Hypertension damages coronary arteries and forces the heart to work harder than it should. It also contributes to atherosclerosis, or hardening of the arteries, and increases the risk of heart attack. This is why it's so important for anyone who has high blood pressure—whether or not they have diabetes—to bring the condition under control. In people with diabetes, hypertension can be even more damaging, since it can contribute to other complications, including diabetic nephropathy and diabetic neuropathy.

### *What Can You Do?*

Fortunately, there are simple measures you can take to lower your blood pressure. The first step is to have your blood pressure checked regularly by a doctor. If you must lose weight, your nutritionist can help you plan a healthy diet that will allow for gradual weight loss. (Losing just a few pounds can reduce blood pressure in many people.) Avoid foods that are high in sodium, which causes fluid retention and raises blood pressure. Also, make sure you stick with your exercise program. Exercise offers many benefits for people with high blood pressure. Regular physical activity will aid you in your weight loss goals and strengthen your cardiovascular system. And working out is a good way to relieve stress, which is a major cause of high blood pressure. (For more information on stress management, see chapter 24.)

If diet and exercise are not enough to help you lower your blood pressure, then your doctor may recommend antihypertension medications. The drugs prescribed for you depend on your unique needs. For example, since certain drugs may cause hypoglycemia, the antihypertension medications prescribed may include ACE inhibitors or calcium channel blockers, which have fewer side effects.

## ATHEROSCLEROSIS

Atherosclerosis occurs when plaque, which is made up of fat and cholesterol, becomes deposited on the walls of the arteries and, to a lesser extent, the veins. This narrows the blood vessels, and eventually makes them hard and inelastic. If measures are not taken to reverse plaque buildup, the blood vessels can become so narrow that they clog easily, preventing the blood from carrying oxygen and nutrients to body tissues.

There are five major risk factors for the development of atherosclerosis: high levels of low-density lipoprotein (LDL) cholesterol, or low levels of high-density lipoprotein (HDL) cholesterol plus high triglycerides, untreated high blood pressure, smoking, poorly controlled diabetes, and a family history of heart disease at a young age.

People with diabetes have an increased risk of developing atherosclerosis, because of the interaction of a number of factors. First, high blood glucose affects the endothelium, the tissue that lines the inner surfaces of the coronary arteries. The cells in the endothelium will malfunction, releasing harmful chemicals that create a sticky surface. This makes the inner walls of the arteries more susceptible to plaque formation. Second, people with diabetes often have higher levels of "bad" LDL cholesterol. Low-density lipoproteins transport cholesterol through the bloodstream to the cells of the body. If LDL is loaded down with more cholesterol than the cells can use, the excess collects on artery walls and forms plaque, which can eventually block arteries. Third, people with diabetes tend to have higher levels of triglycerides, which make up the vast majority of the fat in the foods you eat, and the vast majority of the fat in your body. This is because insulin is needed to efficiently control triglycerides.

When atherosclerosis develops, it affects not only the coronary arteries but all the other arteries. When the arteries in the brain become seriously narrowed, the result is a stroke. The vast majority of strokes are *ischemic,* a term that means loss of blood inflow because of arterial blockage. Ischemic strokes are very similar to heart attacks, but instead of the coronary arteries becoming blocked, the blockage occurs in the brain.

In the legs, serious atheroslcerosis is known as peripheral vascular disease. Peripheral vascular disease is an underlying factor in the development of many of the lower leg and foot problems associated with diabetes. As the plaque builds up, blood flow to the lower legs and feet is decreased.

## WHAT CAN YOU DO?

You can greatly reduce your risk of atherosclerosis by controlling your blood glucose, cholesterol, and triglyceride levels, keeping your blood pressure within a healthy range, and losing weight. Your diabetes treatment program, which should include a healthy meal plan and a program of regular exercise, will enable you to achieve these goals. By including low-fat, high-fiber foods in your diet, you can significantly lower the level of fat in your blood. Research has shown that fiber binds with certain substances that would normally result in the production of cholesterol, and eliminates these substances from the body. In this way, a high-fiber diet helps lower blood cholesterol levels, reducing the risk of cardiovascular disease.

Also, it's important to avoid habits that increase the risk of atherosclerosis, such as smoking. Of course, it is advisable for anyone who smokes to kick the habit, because smoking increases the risk of developing a number of degenerative diseases. However, smoking is especially dangerous for people who have diabetes, because insulin resistance is higher in smokers.

If you are unable to sufficiently lower your LDL cholesterol and triglyceride levels, even despite your best efforts, your physician may prescribe medications that can help. Examples of such medications include atorvastatin (Lipitor), gemfibrozil (Lopid), and simvastatin (Zocor).

In many cases, lifestyle modification, combined with prescription medications (if necessary), is enough to reduce the risk of atherosclerosis by controlling blood cholesterol and triglyceride levels. However, there are instances in which more aggressive medical interventaion may be necessary. For example, if the blood vessels have already narrowed significantly, or if they are blocked, surgery may be the next step. There are a few different procedures that can effectively clear blood vessels and improve circulation. *Balloon angioplasty* is the most common type of angioplasty procedure. For this procedure, a thin tube is guided into the clogged artery, and then a balloon is inflated to push the plaque against the artery wall, which opens up the artery. The balloon is then deflated and withdrawn. Another type of angioplasty procedure is an *arthrectomy.* In this case, instead of pushing the plaque against the wall of the artery, the plaque is scraped off and removed from the area. Additionally, laser surgery can be used to melt away blockages in blood vessels.

When a coronary artery is more severely blocked, bypass surgery may be the best treatment option. Coronary bypass surgery requires moving part of a larger artery from the chest wall or a leg vein, and attaching it above and below the blocked blood vessel. This restores proper circulation by creating a "detour" around the blocked artery, allowing the blood to bypass the blockage by flowing through the new blood vessel.

## Eye Disorders

Vision impairment is a frequent chronic complication of diabetes. In fact, diabetes is the second leading cause of adult blindness. Temporary changes in vision due to the fluctuation of blood sugar levels is common in diabetes, and can be reversed when blood glucose is brought under control. However, high blood sugar over the long-term can cause damage to the tiny blood vessels that supply the retina of the eye, resulting in a condition known as diabetic retinopathy.

The retina is the part of the eye that interprets visual images. It is located in the back of the eye, and contains layers of nerve cells that are sensitive to light. Diabetic retinopathy involves dilation of, and small hemorrhages in, the blood vessels of the retina. If left unchecked, these hemorrhages can scar and pull on the retina, which can cause blindness.

There are two types of retinopathy. In the milder form, known as *non-*

*proliferative retinopathy,* high blood sugar levels damage the delicate blood vessels that nourish the retina. This may cause the blood vessels to become weak or close off, and leak blood, fluid, or fat into the fluid surrounding the retina. If the leakage affects the macula (the part of the eye where vision is sharpest), then the result is blurred vision.

*Proliferative retinopathy* is less common than the nonproliferative form, but it is more serious. In this case, as the delicate small blood vessels in the eye become blocked, new blood vessels form—or proliferate—in that area. In other parts of the body, the formation of new blood vessels can be beneficial, but proliferation can cause severe damage in the eyes. The new blood vessels are fragile and can rupture easily—during exercise, or even while sleeping, especially if high blood pressure is a problem. When they rupture, blood leaks into the fluid portion of the eye located in front of the retina. This blocks light coming into the eye, and thus impairs vision. In addition, scar tissue can form on the retina, creating additional problems.

Eye damage may become apparent shortly after diagnosis in people with type 1 diabetes, and most people with this type of diabetes—up to 97 percent—develop some degree of retinopathy after about fifteen years of living with disease. Retinopathy generally occurs approximately five years after diagnosis in people with type 2 diabetes. The extent to which damage occurs depends upon how well diabetes is controlled.

Other eye problems that can result from diabetes include *glaucoma,* a condition in which the pressure inside the eye increases and damages the optic nerve, and *cataracts,* which are opaque particles inside the lens of the eye that cloud vision. Although glaucoma and cataracts can occur in anyone, people with diabetes are twice as likely to develop these conditions as are nondiabetics. And the less effectively blood glucose levels are controlled, the greater the risk of developing these eye disorders.

## WHAT CAN YOU DO?

By taking the necessary steps to manage your diabetes, you can decrease your risk of developing eye disorders. It is important to remember that over time, high blood sugar levels can damage the eyes wihout causing any changes in vision. Initially, diabetic retinopathy may not even be noticeable. In many cases, only an eye specialist is able to detect the earliest changes in the blood vessels in the eye. This is why regular examinations and follow-ups with an eye doctor are essential. Eye disorders are not inevitable. When eye problems are caught early, much can be done to treat them before permanent damage is done.

So what can you do to reduce your chances of developing eye problems like retinopathy? First, take good care of yourself. Stick with your diabetes treatment program to keep your blood sugar level under control, and keep your regular appointments with your treatment team. And be on the alert for any changes in your vision. Call your doctor if you notice symptoms such as light flashes, dark spots, or rings around lights, or if you have any problems with blurry vision. (Changes in vision may not be a sign of serious eye problems, so don't panic. You may be experiencing symptoms because of temporary high or low glucose levels.) Schedule regular, comprehensive eye exams with a qualified physician who specializes in the management of eye disease in people with diabetes. You probably had an eye exam at the time that you were diagnosed, and depending on your age you should more than likely have one yearly thereafter. Schedule yearly eye exams from age thirty on (or if you're under age thirty and have had diabetes for five years or more).

Treatment for retinopathy (primarily proliferative retinopathy) involves a laser procedure called *photocoagulation.* The doctor uses a laser beam to destroy abnormal blood vessels, patch blood vessels that are leaking, and slow the formation of new blood vessels in the retina. This treatment can be helpful in treating proliferative retinopathy and can also reduce macular edema.

If there has been repeated bleeding into the vitreous gel in the eye, or if scars or other debris in the area impair vision, your doctor may recommend a different surgical procedure, called *vitrectomy.* This procedure replaces the vitreous gel in the eye with a clear solution. Vitrectomy is usually considered to be a last resort to save vision in an affected eye when other treatment is not possible.

# Kidney Problems

Diabetic nephropathy is the medical term used to describe kidney disease caused by diabetes. One third of people with type 1 diabetes and 10 to 20 percent of people with type 2 diabetes develop kidney disease after living with diabetes for fifteen years or more. At its extreme, kidney disease may lead to kidney failure, also known as end-stage renal disease, or ESRD. (Diabetes is the most common cause of kidney failure.) People who have diabetes are twenty times more likely to develop end-stage renal disease than are people who do not have diabetes.

So what happens in diabetic nephropathy? To understand how this complication develops, you need to know a little bit about the structure and function of the kidneys. The kidneys maintain the body's internal environment by controlling its fluid and electrolyte levels, and by removing its waste products. Each kidney contains approximately one million microscopic units called *nephrons,* which filter out waste products from the blood. Over long periods of time, high blood sugar levels damage the tiny blood vessels in the kidneys, making them thicker and clogged, and impairing the filtering ability of the nephrons. As a result, they are less able to filter wastes and impurities from the blood properly. Waste products in the bloodstream then build up to harmful levels. At the same time, some of the nutrients and proteins that should remain in the blood leak out of the blood vessels into the urine. The blood vessels in the kidneys can be further damaged by high blood pressure or kidney infections.

In the early stages, kidney disease is usually silent—there may not be any outward signs to warn that the kidneys are not functioning properly. Usually, one of the first signs of nephropathy is swelling, often in the ankles. (Of course, this doesn't mean that any time you have swelling it's because of kidney problems. There may be other reasons for fluid retention that are not at all related to diabetes.) Other signs to watch out for include anemia, fatigue, weakness, and vomiting.

The first diagnostic sign of nephropathy is usually *microalbuminuria,* the abnormal presence of small amounts of protein in the urine. Kidney function can also be evaluated by measuring the concentration in the blood of substances, such as urea, that are normally eliminated from the body by healthy kidneys. X rays and ultrasound scans may also be performed.

## WHAT CAN YOU DO?

The most important thing you can do to prevent nephropathy—or to minimize its effects—is to keep your blood sugar levels under control. Also, you may need to reduce the amount of protein you eat, since a high-protein diet can greatly affect kidney function. Your dietitian or nutritionist can help you incorporate lower-protein foods into your diabetes meal plan.

Because hypertension increases the risk of kidney disorders, take the necessary steps to keep your blood pressure under control. This may include eating more foods that are rich in potassium, calcium, and magnesium—minerals that are essential to blood pressure control. At the same time, avoid excess sodium, which causes fluid retention and raises blood pressure. Losing weight may also help you reduce your blood pressure. If your blood pressure remains high, your doctor may prescribe an ACE inhibitor. These medications are often effective in improving kidney problems and slowing down the progression of kidney disease.

When the kidneys can no longer perform their filtering function, the patient is said to have end-stage renal disease. Diabetes is the leading cause of ESRD in the United States. Kidney transplantation or dialysis are usually the only treatment options when ESRD develops. Let's take a moment to learn a bit more about these two procedures.

### *Dialysis*

Dialysis is a procedure that performs the functions of the failed kidneys. Remember, the kidneys regulate fluid balance in the body and filter waste products from the blood. When the waste products produced by the body each day are not removed from the blood, they begin to accumulate. Usually, dialysis becomes necessary when waste products reach high levels and cause illness.

There are two types of dialysis—*hemodialysis* and *peritoneal dialysis.* During hemodialysis, blood passes from the patient's body through a filter known as a dialysis membrane in the dialysis machine. The filter removes waste products and excess water, and then the filtered blood passes through the machine and back to the patient. Hemodialysis usually takes place in a hemodialysis unit, a building that is equipped with machines for dialysis treatment. Treatments are scheduled three times a week, with each session lasting from about two to four hours.

Peritoneal dialysis uses the patient's own body tissues to filter waste products from the blood. A plastic tube called a dialysis catheter is inserted through the abdominal wall into an area of the abdominal cavity known as the peritonium (hence, *peritoneal* dialysis), and a special fluid is flushed into the peritonium and washes around the intestines. The intestinal walls act as a filter between this fluid and the bloodstream. Then, the fluid—including the waste products—is drained back out of the body. Peritoneal dialysis is performed by the patient. The procedure usually takes about thirty minutes and must be done four or five times a day.

The decision to undergo one type of dialysis over the other is really up to you. Each method has its relative advantages and disadvantages. For example, some people feel more secure undergoing hemodialysis in a hospital setting, under the watchful eye of a trained professional. They may not mind being restricted to the hospital's dialysis schedule. Others prefer the freedom and convenience of peritoneal dialysis, which can be done at home, despite the fact that they are left more on their own.

### *Kidney Transplantation*

The other alternative for people with end-stage renal disease is kidney transplantation. This is a procedure in which a kidney from a healthy person is donated to a person with kidney failure. The healthy kidney performs all of the functions that the two failed kidneys can no longer carry out.

Kidney transplantation is major surgery and requires careful postoperative care. There is always a risk that the body will reject the new kidney. To minimize this risk, it's important for the donor's blood and tissues to closely match those of the person receiving the kidney. This match will help prevent the body's immune system from rejecting the new kidney. Transplants from living relatives often work better than transplants from unrelated donors. To further minimize the risk of rejection, the doctor will prescribe immunosuppressant medications. However, treatment with these drugs may cause side effects. Because they weaken the immune system, immunosuppressants make it easier to get infections.

In some cases, people getting kidney transplants may also be candidates for pancreas transplants. This may be done at the same time that the kidney is transplanted, or in a later operation. When a pancreas is transplanted, it is surgically placed in the lower part of the abdomen. It drains into the bladder. Once the pancreas is connected it should automatically deliver insulin. In essence, therefore, a successful pancreas transplantation "cures" diabetes.

Although this sounds like the easiest way to treat diabetes, it is only used in more extreme cases, and is usually considered only for people who also need a kidney transplant for survival. There are a number of reasons, including the expense of surgery, the postoperative risks, the chance that it won't work, and that there are not nearly as many of these organs available for people with diabetes who would want (or need) them. These reasons make pancreas transplantation—as it is currently done—less desirable than controlling diabetes through other means.

## Nervous System Disorders

The nervous system is responsible for the coordination of the organs and organ systems in the body, and it enables the body to respond to changes in its internal and external environment. Based on its structure, the nervous system can be divided into two major parts: the *central nervous system,* which includes the brain and spinal cord, and the *peripheral nervous system,* which includes the nerves that link the nervous system with all parts of the body. Damage to the peripheral nervous system is a common complication of diabetes.

So far, we only have theories concerning the link between high blood glucose levels and nervous-system damage. Some scientists believe that elevated blood glucose causes inadequate blood supply to the nerves. There is also the possibility that excess glucose directly damages nerve cells, causing them to scar and swell. And some researchers have theorized that high glucose levels distort the chemical balance inside nerves.

Regardless of the exact cause of nervous-system damage, the outcome is generally the same: Damaged nerves are unable to send signals through the body in the way they normally would. These problems can become apparent as digestive disorders, muscle weakness, problems with bowel or bladder control, heart and blood pressure disorders, and sexual problems. However, because these symptoms also have causes that may be entirely unrelated to diabetes, a complete physical examination is necessary to rule out other possible causes.

The symptoms of neuropathy depend on which nerves and what part of the body are affected. Neuropathy may affect many parts of the body, or it may affect a single, specific nerve and part of the body. The most common forms of neuropathy are outlined below.

*Peripheral symmetrical polyneuropathy* damages the nerves of the limbs of both sides of the body, and causes problems in the arms and/or the legs. It usually begins as a tingling or numbness in the toes, and may ultimately result in loss of reflexes, muscle weakness, loss of sensation, problems with balance and coordination, and a tingling, burning, or prickling feeling in the extremities. As sensation is diminished in the toes or feet, there is the danger of additional injury and even infection. This is dangerous because the person with peripheral neuropathy may not even realize there is a problem, and therefore will not intervene to prevent it from worsening.

*Autonomic neuropathy* results from damage to autonomic nervous system, which controls involuntary actions such as heart rate, breathing, and digestion. This type of neuropathy typically becomes apparent as sexual dysfunction, gastrointestinal disorders, including heartburn, nausea, and vomiting, dizziness and blood pressure problems, and problems with urination, such as urinary retention or urinary incontinence. Usually, symptoms of autonomic-nervous-system damage become apparent with signs of peripheral neuropathy.

*Mononeuropathy* (also called *focal neuropathy*) affects specific nerves, most often in the torso, legs, or head. This type of nerve damage results from a sudden loss of blood to a segment of a particular nerve, or a blockage of individual small blood vessels that supply a particular nerve. Symptoms include localized pain, difficulty focusing the eyes, and paralysis on one side of the face (also known as Bell's palsy). Carpal tunnel syndrome, caused by nerve damage in the wrist, is another sign of focal neuropathy.

Neuropathy develops gradually, and may not become apparent for ten or more years after the initial diagnosis of diabetes. The symptoms of mononeuropathy come on more suddenly than those of other neuropathies, and they often disappear spontaneously after a period of several weeks or months. Once damaged, most nerves cannot go back to normal function.

## WHAT CAN YOU DO?

If you haven't already guessed, tight control is the key to avoiding or minimizing the effects of diabetic neuropathy—and prevention begins with good blood glucose control. Of course, the only way to keep your blood sugar level within a target range is to stick with your diabetes care program and keep regular appointments with your treatment team. Also, if you smoke, you need to kick the habit—statistics show that diabetic neuropathy is more common in smokers—and you should certainly limit your alcohol intake, since alcohol can adversely affect nervous-system function. Even if you are not able to prevent neuropathy, keeping your blood sugar level within your target range can help you delay its onset or at least prevent further tissue damage.

There are some measures you can take to alleviate the pain caused by diabetic neuropathy. Some doctors recommend analgesics such as aspirin, acetaminophen, or anti-inflammatory drugs that contain ibuprofen. Capsaicin, a topical cream, is also available. Additionally, amitriptyline or desipramine, which are typically prescribed to help alleviate the emotional symptoms of depression, may be prescribed the help relieve the pain of peripheral neuropathy. The most common side effects of these medications are drowsiness and dry mouth.

# Foot Problems

Leg and foot problems related to diabetes result from damage to the nerves and blood vessels that supply the legs and feet. Loss of sensation due to nerve damage in the feet is the main cause of foot problems in people with diabetes. If you have a loss of feeling in your feet, you cannot rely on pain to warn you of foot injuries. What seems to be a harmless foot problem—dry skin, a blister, or an ingrown toenail—can quickly progress to a more serious injury if you don't take good care of your feet.

Peripheral vascular disease is an underlying factor in the development of many of the lower leg and foot problems associated with diabetes. This disorder is caused by atherosclerosis, the buildup of plaque within the blood vessels. As the plaque builds up, blood flow to the lower legs and feet is decreased. This means that your feet can't get the proper blood and nutrients they need to heal, and infection is more likely to occur, especially if dirt or germs enter an open wound.

## WHAT CAN YOU DO?

Proper foot care is very important for people with diabetes, to prevent any cuts or other injuries that may lead to a more serious problem. The next goal is for any problem that does develop to be caught as early as possible so that aggressive measures can treat the problem quickly in order to prevent it from progressing.

Because poor circulation is an underlying factor in the development of many foot problems associated with diabetes, you'll need do everything you can to keep the blood flowing easily to your lower legs and feet. Of course, your health depends on your ability to keep your blood sugar level under control, and the best way to do this is to stick with your treatment program. Exercise is doubly important, since regular activity strengthens the entire cardiovascular system, which ensures good circulation. Finally, if you're a smoker, it's time to quit. Smoking decreases circulation to the extremities.

So what steps can you take to prevent foot problems, or to keep them from becoming serious if they do develop? The following guidelines will help keep your feet healthy:

- Always protect your feet. Avoid going barefoot, even indoors. Buy comfortable shoes that fit well—they should not be too tight or too loose, or have toes that are too pointed or too narrow. Leather shoes are a good choice because they allow the air to circulate better around your feet. Be sure to wear your shoes with socks or stockings.
- Keep the skin on your feet clean, dry, and healthy. After you wash your feet, pat them dry carefully, since excess moisture can promote the growth of fungus, which can cause athlete's foot and other disorders. To prevent dryness, apply lotion to dry skin after your bath or shower. Avoid applying lotion between the toes, because this can cause athlete's foot.
- File your toenails straight across; toenails that are not trimmed properly can press into adjacent toes and cut the skin. It's best to avoid using scissors or clippers, so you won't cut yourself—any cuts increase the likelihood of infection.
- Before bathing, test the bathwater with your elbow or a bath thermometer to avoid scalding your feet. Remember that you may not be able to detect high temperatures with your feet if you have nerve damage.

Should you develop any foot problems, remember that early intervention is the key to preventing further damage. Look at your feet and examine them thoroughly at least once a day, and also after exercising. You should be looking for cuts or breaks in the skin, bruises, swollen or red areas, calluses, blisters, changes in color, and insect bites. Also, check the temperature of your feet. If they're too cold, this may suggest poor blood circulation; if they're too warm, this may indicate an infection. Immediately report any problems you identify to your doctor or a podiatrist who is experienced in treating people with diabetes. Don't attempt to treat any foot problem by yourself, no matter how minor you may think it is. In addition, have your doctor check your feet at each visit.

Many people with diabetes are frightened about the possibility of amputation in the case of foot problems. Remember that preventing problems before they develop is the most important thing you can do to ensure that you won't have to undergo this type of surgery. And even if foot problems do occur, you can take steps to minimize further injury. So you understand the significance of proper foot care, let's take a quick look at a situation in which amputation might be considered.

If an infection is aggressive—regardless of the treatment you've been receiving—amputation may be considered to keep the infection from spreading. In some cases, poor circulation can cause gangrene, which results from infection by the bacteria clostridia. Because clostridia grows only in the absence of oxygen, poor circulation allows for infection by this kind of bacteria. Gangrene is actually the death of tissue, and it is a breeding ground for infection. Amputation may be required to prevent the spread of infection and extensive tissue damage. Remember, though, that this kind of extreme case can very likely be prevented with proper attention to foot care.

## Skin Problems

Your skin is your body's first line of defense against invasion by germs and the development of infections. Unfortunately, people with diabetes are at increased risk of infection because of nerve damage, which makes repeated injury to the skin more likely. Poor circulation also contributes to the risk of infection, since blood and nutrients can't reach the site of injury to help in the healing process.

In chapter 6, we discussed lipoatrophy and hypertrophy, two skin conditions that result from insulin injections. Lipoatrophy is caused by the loss of fatty tissue under the skin, which appears to be caused by an immune reaction to insulin, and may also result from repeated trauma to the injection site. Hypertrophy is an accumulation of fat cells at the injection site that looks similar to scar tissue. Rotating injection sites is the best way to avoid or alleviate these two conditions. Additionally, bruising may occur at the site where insulin is injected, usually because the needle has nicked a tiny blood vessel. In most cases, this is not a significant problem.

When blood glucose levels are not well controlled, extra urine is produced to rid the body of excess blood glucose. This can lead to dehydration, which can cause dry skin. Autonomic neuropathy may affect the body's sweating mechanisms, and this may also cause the skin to dry out. When the skin is dry, it is more likely to crack or break, allowing bacteria to enter the site and cause infection.

Other skin-related problems that are statistically more likely to occur in people with diabetes include fungal infections, a depigmentation of the skin called vitiligo, and loss of hair on the head, known scientifically as alopecia.

## WHAT CAN YOU DO?

With proper care, skin problems can usually be avoided. The following guidelines will help you keep your skin healthy.

- When you bathe or shower, make sure the water is lukewarm, especially if you have lost sensation in your skin—hot water can dry your skin out and can scald you. Use a mild soap that will not dry your skin.
- After you bathe or shower, dry your skin well, and then apply a light moisturizer to keep your skin soft and prevent skin cracks or breaks.
- Drink plenty of fluids to stay well hydrated.
- Wear clothing that allows better air circulation.
- Protect your skin against the cold. If you must go out in very cold weather, dress warmly.

Sores that do not heal, redness, swelling, pus, heat, and pain may all signal the presence of an infection. If you notice any of these symptoms, let your doctor know. Rashes, itching, or other signs of infection should also be reported, as well as blisters or bumps.

Although skin problems can be annoying and can increase the chances for infection, usually the skin is not seriously affected by diabetes. In many cases the problems clear up by themselves or they simply become bothersome or inconvenient rather than dangerous.

## Tooth Problems

Although it's important for everyone to take care of their teeth, it's especially important for people with diabetes. There is an increased likelihood of bacteria formation because of the higher glucose levels in your body. Your saliva may be sweeter than normal if you have higher glucose levels. This may lead to increased bacteria in your mouth, which can increase your chances for gum infections. And, as you already know, it's important to fight infections, because diabetes makes it more difficult to fight them off.

### WHAT CAN YOU DO?

Brush regularly (at least twice a day) and floss in order to remove bacteria from between your teeth. Watch for signs that should be immediately reported to your dentist, including swollen, red, tender, or bleeding gums, gums that seem to have pulled away from your teeth, and any other changes in your teeth, tongue, or breath. Make sure that your teeth are professionally cleaned and checked regularly—at least every six months.

## An Uncomplicated Conclusion

Although complications can be serious (and scary), there's a lot you can do to prevent them or to minimize their effects. Learn as much as you can, make sure that you get up-to-date information about treatment for any complications that you may experience, work with your treatment team, and—most important—don't stick your head in the sand. Be aware of potential problems . . . and act on them.

# CHAPTER TWELVE

# Pregnancy and Diabetes

Until about twenty-five years ago, women with type 1 and type 2 diabetes were often discouraged from attempting pregnancy because of the health risks involved. Fortunately, the development of new tests and new theories about managing diabetes have made it possible for women with diabetes to plan to have a family. We now know that the key to a healthy pregnancy is tight blood sugar control—before and during pregnancy.

Before we begin our discussion, let me remind you that gestational diabetes is different from pregnancy in type 1 and type 2 diabetes. As you'll recall from chapter 1, gestational diabetes results from changes in the levels and types of hormones produced during pregnancy. Women with gestational diabetes actually have plenty of insulin in their blood. The problem is that insulin's action is partially blocked by pregnancy hormones secreted by the placenta.

Because gestational diabetes occurs during the course of the pregnancy and disappears after the baby is born, some of the information presented in this chapter—for example, the material on prepregnancy planning—will not apply to women with this condition. However, gestational diabetes poses the same health risks to the mother and baby as type 1 and type 2 diabetes, so the treatment plan outlined here will benefit women with any of the three types of diabetes.

## What Are the Risks?

Today, a pregnant woman with diabetes can look forward to having a healthy baby. But there still is an element of risk for both the mother and her child. This is especially true if the mother-to-be doesn't manage her diabetes properly. Women with poorly controlled diabetes have a greater chance of giving birth to babies that are abnormally large, approaching ten pounds or more. This condition—known medically as macrosomia—occurs because the extra sugar in the mother's blood crosses the placenta to the developing baby, which in turn causes the baby's blood sugar to rise. As a result, the baby's body produces more insulin, causing the extra sugar to be stored as fat.

There is also some evidence that women with poorly controlled diabetes are more likely to give birth to babies with serious birth defects, such as neural tube defects, and have a greater chance of preterm delivery and even miscarriage or stillbirth.

Women who do not take steps to control their blood sugar are also at greater risk of developing *pregnancy-induced hypertension* (PIH). PIH affects both the mother and her unborn child. The condition constricts blood flow to the uterus, which results in the baby receiving less oxygen and nutrients. Also, PIH may cause the placenta to separate from the wall of the uterus before delivery, resulting in bleeding and shock. Left untreated, PIH may progress to preeclampsia, which is characterized by high blood pressure, protein in the urine, sudden weight gain, and swelling of the face and hands.

## What About Genetics?

You may be concerned that you will pass diabetes on to your child. Research suggests that there are many different factors that determine whether children will develop diabetes, including whether one or both parents have diabetes, what type of diabetes they have, and what family history of diabetes exists. Some studies have shown that children born to parents with type 1 diabetes are at slightly greater risk of developing type 1 diabetes than children of parents who do not have diabetes. However, the risk varies depending on whether it is the mother or the father who has diabetes.

The risk of the baby developing diabetes also varies based on the age of the mother. Mothers below age twenty-five seem to have the greater likelihood of having children born with diabetes than mothers older than twenty-five. Although there is no guarantee that your child will develop diabetes, it can be a good idea to get genetic counseling before you get pregnant in order to determine what the risks might be.

## Before Conception

The best chance for a normal pregnancy will occur when diabetes is brought under control *before* planned conception. Most women do not know they are pregnant until two to four weeks after conception. But during the first six weeks of pregnancy, the baby's organs are forming—and your blood sugar levels during these early weeks affect the baby's growth and development. Because high blood sugar levels during these early weeks can lead to birth defects, you need to plan your pregnancy.

If you are going to try to conceive, discuss your decision with your physician and other members of your health-care team. Health professionals can assess your condition and tell you if pregnancy is advisable, or if you should wait until your diabetes is brought under better control. Generally, women with diabetes who are planning conception should bring their diabetes under tight control three to six months before becoming pregnant.

What if you doctor advises against pregnancy at this time? If you are going to be sexually active, then you'll need to use an effective form of birth control. Your options include birth control pills, intrauterine devices, and barrier methods (condoms or diaphragm plus spermicide). The risk of unplanned pregnancies with any of these birth control options are reduced as long as the techniques are used correctly. Talk with your doctor to find out which method will work best for you.

Be aware that oral diabetes medications can cause birth defects, so if you're using any of these medications to control type 2 diabetes, you'll need to switch to insulin at least a month *before* you get pregnant. This will give you time to become accustomed to giving yourself injections, and to learn how to balance insulin with diet and exercise.

Certain immunosuppressive drugs should also be discontinued prior to conception. Discuss any medications being used with your treatment team to determine which may need to be stopped, and how long you need to wait before trying to conceive.

## Ensuring a Healthy Pregnancy

After you become pregnant, you'll have to see your physician and your obstetrician much more often than a woman who does not have diabetes. You will also have to be more diligent about controlling your blood sugar levels than you were before your pregnancy. This means that you'll need to make some changes in your diabetes treatment program, such as adjusting to insulin injections, checking your blood sugar levels more frequently, testing daily for ketones, and modifying your diet and exercise program. The following material is meant to provide an overview of the types of changes you should expect to make during pregnancy. Your treatment team will be able to provide you with specific guidelines that are suited to your unique needs.

### ADJUSTING TO INSULIN INJECTIONS

During pregnancy, a woman's body requires more insulin—regardless of whether diabetes is a factor. Why? The body's ability to process carbohydrates changes during pregnancy to ensure an adequate supply of glucose for the developing baby. In women who do not have diabetes, the body naturally produces more insulin to balance blood sugar levels. This is not the case for pregnant women who have diabetes.

Remember, when the body doesn't have enough insulin to enable glucose—its main source of energy—to enter the cells, it is forced to use body fat as an energy source. Ketones are byproducts of fat breakdown that can accumulate in the bloodstream and spill over into the urine. Diabetic ketoacidosis occurs when the body chemistry becomes acidic because of the buildup of ketones. It can develop quickly, and it is life threatening.

As mentioned earlier, if you have type 2 diabetes and you have been taking oral diabetes medications to manage your condition, you'll need to begin taking insulin instead. And even if you are accustomed to taking insulin—for example, if you have type 1 diabetes—your doctor will probably prescribe a larger dose to be taken more often during your pregnancy. If have gestational diabetes, a healthy diet combined with a program of regular exercise may be enough to keep your blood sugar under control. However, if you have trouble managing your diabetes despite your diet and exercise plan, you will need to begin taking insulin.

## BLOOD GLUCOSE MONITORING

Because tight glucose control is so important during pregnancy, you will have to monitor your blood sugar levels much more frequently to make sure you're staying within your target range. Most doctors recommend a fasting blood glucose level of 60 to 100 mg/dl for pregnant women with diabetes. The suggested range one to two hours after eating is between 100 and 140 mg/dl.

## TESTING FOR KETONES

Urine testing for ketones is a very important part of diabetes management for women with type 1 diabetes during pregnancy. Because this was not part of your management program before pregnancy, daily testing for ketones may take some adjustment. You should test your urine for ketones each morning before you eat or take insulin. If ketones are present in your urine two days in a row—even if blood sugar is normal or close to normal—call your doctor. This may be a sign that you are developing diabetic ketoacidosis.

## EATING FOR TWO

Nutritional planning is essential during pregnancy. Because of potential weight gain, you will need sufficient calories to support both your own strength and the growth of the baby. Your doctor will determine your nutritional and weight goals depending on a variety of factors, including your size, your prepregnancy weight, your current weight, and whether or not you have hypertension.

In addition to eating healthy to control your diabetes, you'll have to eat nutrient-packed foods that will help you meet your nutritional requirements during pregnancy. Remember, you'll be eating for two! Because you have diabetes, you should already be eating a healthy, low-fat diet that includes lots of fresh, whole foods. While you're pregnant, you'll have to be careful to take in an adequate supply of essential nutrients such as protein, which is vital to your baby's growth, and calcium, which helps build strong baby bones. Additionally, supplements of folic acid—an important B vitamin—are strongly recommended for women who are pregnant or planning to become pregnant. Scientific evidence shows that folic acid can prevent neural tube defects in many babies.

Your dietitian will help you devise an eating plan that will ensure good health for you *and* your baby.

## EXERCISING

You already know about all the benefits exercise has to offer people with diabetes. Well, pregnancy is no reason to stop exercising. In fact, regular physical activity is just as essential, if not more so. Exercise will help you control your blood sugar levels, which will minimize the risk of complications during pregnancy. It will enable you to maintain a healthy weight, because you burn extra calories and fat. It will increase your strength and stamina, and will better prepare you for labor and delivery.

So how much should you exercise? In general, it's not a good idea to start a new, strenuous exercise program during pregnancy. Most experts agree that moderate aerobic activities, such as walking, swimming, and low-impact aerobics, offer many benefits and few risks for expectant mothers. However, if you have any complications related to diabetes—high blood pressure, eye, kidney, or heart problems, damage to small or large blood vessels, nerve damage—certain exercises may not be appropriate for you. To be certain that you're doing what's best for you and your baby, you'll need to discuss exercise options with your treatment team.

Because of the potential for your blood sugar levels to decline as a result of exercise, you must guard against hypoglycemia. Research suggests that hypoglycemia does not affect the fetus directly. However, it can certainly affect the mother, and because you're carrying the baby it is still something to be avoided. In order to determine how exercise affects your blood glucose level, you should always check your blood sugar before you exercise. You may need to have a snack prior to or during exercise, or immediately after finishing your exercise routine, to prevent hypoglycemia.

## PROTECTING YOUR EYES

There is an increased possibility that eye problems can develop in women with diabetes during pregnancy, so it's very important to have your eyes checked by an ophthalmologist. If you've had retinopathy prior to pregnancy, your doctor must evaluate your condition and determine whether or not it's wise for you to become pregnant.

It is usually recommended that women with diabetes have their eyes checked two or three times during their pregnancy. Early detection is the key to proper treatment, because the doctor can begin treating any minor problems before they develop into more serious concerns.

## USING MEDICATIONS

As we've already discussed, it's a good idea to avoid most medications during pregnancy. But this is not always possible. Don't take decisions regarding medication and pregnancy lightly. And don't take decisions into your own hands. That's what you have a doctor for, right?

What if you discover that you're pregnant while you're on medication? Your doctor may want you to stop the medication as soon as possible. It's okay to abruptly stop taking some medicines. But discontinuing the use of certain medications very suddenly can be dangerous indeed. Whether you should continue medication, stop it, or even consider pregnancy is a matter that you'll want to discuss with your family and your treatment team.

# Tests During Pregnancy

During your pregnancy, you will undergo a number of different tests to ensure that your baby is developing properly. Some tests are used routinely in pregnancy to determine fetal position and the sex of the baby, or to detect fetal abnormalities. Other tests are used in certain cases of pregnancy complications. Make sure you understand all the risks and benefits involved before agreeing to or rejecting a procedure. If you don't feel comfortable about taking a particular test, continue to ask questions and to request explanations until the doctor has eased your concern.

Among the common tests used in pregnancy are ultrasound, amniocentesis, alpha-fetoprotein (AFP) screening, the nonstress test, and the oxytocin challenge test (OCT).

## ULTRASOUND

A form of ultrasound used in pregnancy is the sonogram, which uses intermittent sound waves. The sound waves are directed into the woman's abdomen, with an outline of the baby, placenta, and other structures involved in pregnancy transmitted to a video screen. A sonogram is often used to determine fetal position, to estimate the maturity of the baby, or to confirm a multiple pregnancy.

## AMNIOCENTESIS

Amniocentesis is used to detect abnormalities in the baby. The test is performed by administering a local anesthetic, then withdrawing a samply of amniotic fluid using a long needle inserted through the abdominal and uterine walls. A complete chromosomal analysis is done on the sample to detect the presence of Down's syndrome or other genetic abnormalities. Amniocentesis can also be used to determine the sex of the baby.

### ALFA-FETOPROTEIN SCREENING

Alfa-fetoprotein screening is a blood test performed between the fifteenth and eighteenth weeks of pregnancy to screen for fetal abnormalities. AFP is a protein produced by the baby. A high level in the expectant mother's blood indicates a possible neural tube defect, such as spina bifida or anencephaly. A low level may indicate Down's syndrome.

### NONSTRESS TEST

The nonstress test is a very reliable noninvasive test that measures fetal heart rate in response to fetal activity as observed on a fetal monitor. The expectant mother is placed on an electric fetal monitor and a baseline heart rate is noted. The women is given a control to push when she feels the baby move. The control places a mark on the readout.

An increase in the fetal heart rate indicates fetal well-being. If the result is negative, additional testing is usually performed.

### OXYTOCIN CHALLENGE TEST

The oxytocin challenge test, also known as a stress test, helps determine how well the baby will undergo the stress of labor. Oxytocin is a medicine that causes uterine contractions. The mother-to-be is given oxytocin intravenously until she has contractions three to four minutes apart for a full half hour. At the same time, the baby's heart rate is electronically monitored to check the effects of the contractions. If the fetal heart rate appears abnormal, the doctor may recommend a cesarean birth, which causes less stress on the baby.

## After Delivery

In uncomplicated cases, most women with diabetes can deliver close to their due date. To be safe, an obstetrician may deliver a baby slightly before the due date by inducing labor or by cesarean birth.

Most babies born to women with diabetes require extra care immediately following delivery. This doesn't mean that you didn't do a good job of managing your diabetes during pregnancy. Instead, it is done to ensure a close watch and quick treatment for any problems that may develop, such as low blood sugar.

## Breast-feeding

If you are planning to breast-feed your baby, you'll be happy to know that breast-feeding is perfectly safe for mothers with diabetes. In fact, breast-feeding appears to offer some advantages over bottle feeding. For example, experts say that breast-feeding causes the uterus to return to its prepregnant state faster. Breast milk is an ideal food for your baby—it's packed with nutrients, and it also contains some of your own antibodies, which will help your baby fight off illness. And some research suggests that babies who are breast-fed for at least three months have a lower incidence of type 1 diabetes.

Be aware, however, that for all of its advantages, breast-feeding offers one disadvantage for women with diabetes. Because your body requires more energy to produce breast milk, your blood sugar levels may be more difficult to predict. Therefore, if you decide to breast-feed your baby, you will need to monitor your blood sugar level more frequently, and to make sure that you take insulin exactly as it is prescribed for you. To guard against hypoglycemia, you may want to have a snack before or during breast-feeding. You should also keep a fast-acting sugar nearby in case your blood sugar levels drops.

## Are You Pacified?

Pregnancy is a joyous, exciting time for the mother-to-be and her family and friends. For women with diabetes, however, pregnancy can be risky. Because of the increased chances of birth defects, pregnancy-induced hypertension, and other complications, women with diabetes must be extra cautious when it comes to self-care.

If you and your partner are planning a pregnancy, discuss the decision with your doctor. Be open and honest in your discussion, and express any of your concerns about the potential risks of pregnancy. Make sure you fully understand all that's involved in ensuring a healthy pregnancy. Take all these factors into consideration and then—good luck!

## CHAPTER THIRTEEN

# Dealing with Sick Days

As you make the adjustment to living with diabetes, you'll find that self-care becomes easier. Monitoring your blood glucose will become an integral part of your daily routine, just like getting dressed in the morning or brushing your teeth. Taking insulin or other diabetes medications will not seem like such a daunting task as you become more adept at anticipating how your body will respond. Choosing healthy foods that fit easily into your diet plan will be like second nature, and you may even find yourself looking forward to your daily workout. How is all of this possible? It's just a matter of accepting your new lifestyle—and all of the responsibilities that come with it—and incorporating the components of your treatment program into the routine of your everyday life. It's all about familiarity.

But what happens in situations that take you out of your daily routine? Let's talk about sick days. Even ordinary illnesses such as colds and flu require extra-special care. This chapter will cover the special care you require and the things you must remember to do when you're not feeling well.

# What Happens When You're Sick?

When you get sick, your body releases hormones to fight the illness. This is a normal reaction, and one that is meant to be beneficial. Unfortunately, for people with diabetes this defense mechanism can have some troubling consequences. You see, the hormones released to fight illnesses—even minor ailments like colds—cause an increased release of stored glucose from the liver. This is the body's way of supplying more energy to overcome the illness. But these same hormones may also increase insulin resistance, so your cells can't make good use of the extra energy. In fact, you'll probably feel even more fatigued when this happens.

If blood sugar is allowed to rise unchecked, your body may begin to rely more on fat for energy. And as stored fat is burned at increasing rates, toxic substances called ketones are produced. In people with type 1 diabetes, ketone production can cause diabetic ketoacidosis; in people with type 2 diabetes, it may lead to hyperglycemic hyperosmolar syndrome. (Refer back to chapter 10 for a detailed discussion of these two conditions.)

Because any illness can be potentially dangerous for people with diabetes, it's essential that you speak with your doctor and get specific instructions about self-care during sick days. You will need to know how often you should monitor your blood glucose when you're sick, when you will need to take more or less of your insulin or diabetes medication, which over-the-counter medications are safe for you to use, and—if you have type 1 diabetes—when you should check for ketones in your urine. By getting all the important information *before* you get sick, you will be prepared to take good care of yourself.

# Recommendations for Sick Days

When you are developing a cold, flu, or other illness, your blood sugar levels will often be higher than usual because your body is trying to ward off infection.

## MONITOR YOUR BLOOD SUGAR

You should monitor your blood sugar four to five times a day when you're ill. The best times to check your blood sugar level is before each meal, before bedtime, and once during the night. Write down the times you checked your blood glucose, and the results, and be prepared to give this information to your doctor, if necessary. Although you may feel too tired or ill to be vigilant about tracking your blood sugar, remember that there may be serious consequences (such as ketoacidosis or HHS) if your blood sugar rises too high. If your blood glucose is over 240 mg/dl, you should also test for ketones in your urine.

## CONTINUE TAKING YOUR MEDICATION

Never stop taking your diabetes medication or decrease your dose when you are sick, unless your doctor advises you to do so. Even if you can't eat, you still must take your medication to counteract the extra glucose that your body releases to fight illness. Keep the lines of communication open with your doctor—he or she can tell you whether you need to increase or decrease your dosage. Some people with type 2 diabetes may need to take insulin while they're sick, but this should be temporary.

## KEEP EATING

Try to stick with your regular eating plan when you're sick. If you are unable to follow your normal diet because you are nauseated or vomiting, supplement food intake by sipping beverages that contain sugar, to avoid hypoglycemia. Easy-to-digest foods that can supplement your usual diet include soups, gelatin with sugar, juice, eggs, and similar foods. If you are vomiting, sip a caffeine-free—not diet—soft drink or any drink containing sugar. Speak with your dietitian about good foods and drinks for sick days before you get sick, so you'll be prepared to accommodate any changes in your appetite when you become ill.

### DRINK FLUIDS

It's always important to drink plenty of fluids during periods of illness, even for people who don't have diabetes. Try to drink at least eight ounces of fluid without sugar every hour during the day to prevent dehydration. This is especially important if you are vomiting or have diarrhea, because your body is losing more fluids.

### BE CAUTIOUS ABOUT USING OVER-THE-COUNTER MEDICATIONS

Many over-the-counter medications affect blood glucose control. Be careful with any over-the-counter medication that you may consider taking to try to feel better when you're sick. Read all labels and instructions carefully, and avoid products that contain sugar, alcohol, or epinephrine. For example, cough or cold remedies that are labeled decongestants may contain ingredients such as pseudoephedrine that increase blood glucose levels and blood pressure. Other medications, such as cough or cold remedies, may contain sugar and even alcohol. Find out what active and inactive ingredients are in any medication that you're considering taking. Most important, make sure you discuss these medications with your treatment team.

### TAKE A BREAK FROM EXERCISE

When you are sick, it's very important to rest and conserve your energy so that your body can fight the illness. Also, exercising when you are sick can cause your blood sugar level to rise.

## Know When to Contact Your Treatment Team

Knowing when to call your doctor is an important part of being prepared for sick days. That's why it's a good idea to talk to your doctor before you have to face the special challenges that sick days present. Ask your doctor what kinds of symptoms necessitate a call, and what degree of illness requires his or her attention. Usually, it's important to call your doctor if:

- You do not improve in one day.
- You have vomiting or diarrhea that occurs more than once.
- Your blood glucose level is below 60 mg/dl.
- You're taking insulin and you experience a hypoglycemic reaction.
- Your blood glucose level is higher than 240 mg/dl.
- You experience symptoms of hyperglycemia, including extreme thirst, extreme hunger, dry mouth, or a fruity odor on your breath.
- You experience mental confusion or disorientation.
- You are sleepier than usual, or you are becoming progressively weaker.
- You experience any difficulty breathing
- You have chest or stomach pains.

If you have any doubts about what you should be doing to take care of yourself during your illness, don't hesitate to call your doctor for advice. Remember, your treatment team is there to help you successfully manage your diabetes day by day.

## Here's to Your Health

Coping with diabetes includes good self-care during sick days. Sure, this is more difficult than managing your diabetes when you're feeling well, and it may be a little scary the first time you find yourself out of your regular groove. But if you know what to do, and you take proper care of yourself, you'll get back up to speed in no time.

## CHAPTER FOURTEEN

# Preparing for Travel

Mel is a fifty-five-year-old attorney. One reason he has always enjoyed working hard at his job is that it provides him with an income sufficient to take his family on luxurious annual vacations all over the globe. However, since he was diagnosed with diabetes, Mel has not taken any trips at all. Why? You see, Mel is afraid that he won't be able to stick to his diabetes management program or find a doctor who can help him if he travels, so he doesn't want to go away from home. But it doesn't have to be this way!

People with diabetes can travel to almost any corner of the globe. However, going away from home *doesn't* mean you can take a vacation from your diabetes treatment program. In fact, because you'll be taken out of your everyday routine, you'll need to be even more careful about what you eat, when you eat, and how often you monitor your blood sugar. Plus, you will need to fit in some time for exercise. Remember, taking good care of yourself will not impinge on your vacation plans. Quite the contrary! Sticking to your treatment program when you are away will help you to have a more enjoyable vacation, because you'll be minimizing the risk of falling ill.

Let's explore some of the ways you can prepare for a comfortable—and safe—trip away from home.

## Plan Ahead

You don't have to restrict your travel plans just because you have diabetes. With proper planning and preparation, you can go anywhere you want, by plane, train, automobile, or cruise ship. The following guidelines will help you better prepare yourself for your travels.

### SCHEDULE A COMPLETE PHYSICAL

Before you leave for your trip, you should schedule an appointment with your health-care team for a complete physical. This will ensure that your diabetes is under control, and that you're in good health to make your upcoming trip.

Find out if you need to get any immunization shots prior to your trip. Depending on where you're traveling, there's a very real possibility that you may need to be immunized. Because of the chance that the shots may cause your blood sugar to become temporarily uncontrolled, you should get your immunization shots at least a month before you depart. This way, you'll have plenty of time to bring your diabetes back under control.

### GET A SIGNED LETTER FROM YOUR DOCTOR

Ask for a letter signed by your doctor stating that you have diabetes. The letter should certify that you must carry insulin or oral diabetes medication, syringes, and other supplies with you. To be safe, carry with you prescriptions for your medications with the generic name of the medications identified. Doctors and pharmacists in other countries may not recognize American brand names, so if you have the generic name on hand, you'll be ready if you need to buy medication during your trip.

### RESEARCH YOUR DESTINATION

Research your destination to find out how to get medical care. Try to get the names of doctors, hospitals, or even affiliates of the American Diabetes

Association in the area to which you will be traveling. The International Association for Medical Assistance to Travelers can be of great help if you're trying to learn more about medical care abroad. Call 716-754-4883.

## PACK EXTRA MEDICATION AND SUPPLIES

Bring more than enough diabetes medication and supplies with you in case your return home is delayed. You'll want to make sure that you have an ample supply of syringes (if you use insulin), as well as the materials you need for blood glucose testing and urine testing for ketones.

Ask your physician to write up extra prescriptions for your medications and other supplies. It's very important that you know exactly which type of syringe you use, since this can vary, especially in other countries. And be aware that different types and strengths of insulin are available in different countries. The type of insulin you normally take may not be available.

Carry all of your medications and supplies with you in one bag. This includes your diabetes medications and glucagon, as well as over-the-counter remedies for colds, diarrhea, and nausea. Plus, you'll probably want to bring along some rubbing alcohol and cotton swabs. Although this may involve a little more carry-on luggage than you would like, the peace of mind you'll have knowing that you're prepared is well worth it.

## PACK OVER-THE-COUNTER MEDICATIONS

Nobody likes getting sick, especially on vacation. But if you're traveling far from home, there's a greater chance that you'll experience diarrhea or nausea. Travelers are often warned not to drink tap water when they travel to certain countries, and to be careful trying new and exotic foods. While it's important for all travelers to heed these warnings, people with diabetes need to be especially cautious about what they eat and drink. That's because nausea and/or diarrhea can throw blood sugar levels out of control. To prevent the occurrence of either of these reactions, stick with bottled beverages instead of tap water. And, of course, make sure you pack over-the-counter medications to treat gastrointestinal upset, so that you can prevent any problems that may occur from becoming worse.

### REQUEST SPECIAL MEALS IN ADVANCE

If you are traveling by plane, you can request special meals that will fit easily into your diet plan. This usually needs to be done at least twenty-four hours in advance of your flight. However, you may find that regular meals are more appealing and filling than their diabetic alternatives, which is sometimes as simple as fruit and crackers. Check with your nutritionist to see if regular meals will fit into your diet plan.

Many cruise ships have accommodations for people with special physical needs. Speak to your travel agent or a representative of the cruise line several weeks in advance if you wish to request special meals. Do remember, however, that you *can* eat many of the foods that your companions will be enjoying—you just need to be smart about the foods that you choose, and make sure you eat appropriate portions.

## Self-Care Away from Home

If you're smart about packing and plan ahead, you'll have little to worry about—wherever you decide to travel. Remember, though, that if you're going to relax and have fun, you can't afford to take a break from your treatment program. The travel tips provided below will help you stay on track.

### KEEP MEDICATIONS AND SUPPLIES WITH YOU AT ALL TIMES

Carry your medication, supplies, testing materials, and glucagon in a carry-on bag, rather than packing them in with the rest of your luggage. Why? Well, for one thing, if your bags end up in Denver when you're flying to Fort Lauderdale, you'll be without some of the essential components of your treatment program. If you carry your supplies with you, you'll have what you need when you need it, whether you're traveling by bus, train, or plane. Remember also that it's important to protect insulin and other medications, as well as glucose testing strips, from extreme temperatures, since heat and cold can ruin them. Who knows what the temperature's like where your luggage is stored?

If you must take injections during a flight, put less air (possibly only half as much) into the insulin bottle as you normally would. In-flight cabin pressure is lower, so you don't have to inject as much air into the insulin bottle when you draw up insulin.

## TAKE TIME ZONES INTO ACCOUNT

If you are going to be traveling across time zones, ask your doctor or diabetes educator for advice on how to adjust your medication. If you're traveling east, for example, your day will be shorter because you're going to lose time. As a result, you'll need less insulin. When you travel west, on the other hand, your day will be longer. As such, you'll need more insulin. If you're worried that you won't be able to make the proper adjustments, check your blood glucose more frequently and readjust your dose as necessary.

## CARRY A SNACK WITH YOU

Although you should continue to eat every four to five hours, as usual, be prepared in case a meal is delayed. (After all, even the best laid travel plans often go astray!) Carry an emergency snack pack with you wherever you go. You should also pack a substantial snack—a piece of fruit or cheese and crackers, for example—to tide you over, as well as some form of quick-acting glucose in case your blood sugar drops too low.

## IDENTIFY YOURSELF

It's always a good idea to travel with complete identification, because this will make it easier for others to help you if for some reason you cannot help yourself. The Medic Alert bracelet is accepted worldwide as identification for people with medical conditions. In addition, carry an identification card with you. Include complete details about your diabetes, a list of symptoms that require treatment, the type of medication you require, and the names of your physician and other members of your health-care team. The card should also list contact telephone numbers in case a friend or family member needs to be contacted.

If you're going to a foreign country, you may want to have the information on your card translated in the language of that country. You may need help with this, if you're not fluent in that particular language. Try checking with a foreign-language teacher at a local school. Or you can contact a representative of an airline that travels to that country. Representatives who speak the language will probably be willing to translate for you.

If you're not traveling with family members or friends who know about diabetes and what to do if there is an emergency, make sure that you inform someone about your condition. For example, if you're going to be touring with a group, you might want to let the group leader know that you have diabetes, and explain what to do in case you have an insulin reaction.

## DON'T FORGET TO EXERCISE!

Make sure that you include regular exercise wherever you go. For example, if you travel on a train or a plane, get up periodically and walk around. If you travel by bus or car, take frequent breaks—every one to two hours—to stretch your legs.

If you are going to be more active than usual, be prepared for your blood glucose level to fluctuate. Vacationing often includes lots of touring and sight-seeing, and can really cause your blood sugar to drop. Your doctor or diabetes educator can help you determine how your diet and/or medications should be adjusted to compensate for extra activity.

## WEAR COMFORTABLE WALKING SHOES

Many people like to "see the sights" when they're vacationing—and this often requires a lot of walking! To protect your feet against blisters and cuts, wear cotton socks and comfortable walking shoes. And remember to take good care of your feet at the end of a long day of sight-seeing. Apply lotion to dry skin to minimize the risk of cracks. Examine your feet closely for cuts, blisters, insect bites, and bruises, and look for any areas that are red, hot, swollen, or tender. (For more tips on foot care, refer to chapter 11.)

### PREVENT SUNBURN

Depending on where you travel, sunburn can be a very real possibility. Sunburn can stress your body and increase your blood sugar level. If you're going to be working on your tan, make sure you wear a strong sunblock and gradually increase your time in the sun. Try to avoid being out in the sun during the midday hours, when the sun's rays are most powerful. If you'll be out in the sunshine when you're sight-seeing, apply sunblock before you go outside, and wear a hat while you're in the sun. If it's not too hot, you may want to consider wearing long pants and a long-sleeved shirt, as well.

## All Aboard!

If you haven't traveled recently, you may want to build up your confidence by taking short trips first. Taking a three-month trip around the world might be a bit much! Start with a couple of day trips, then weekend trips, working your way up to short-distance, week-long excursions. Expanding your travel activities slowly is a good way to develop your confidence.

A lot of information has been provided here—mostly precautionary, but nevertheless realistic and sensible. You may need extra time to prepare for your vacation, but this extra preparation will enable you to enjoy a wonderful vacation, just like any other globe-trotter. Don't forget to send me a postcard!

## CHAPTER FIFTEEN

# Managing Pain

Ouch! (Just getting you ready for this chapter!) Is diabetes painful? It can be, especially if you're experiencing diabetic neuropathy. But the good news is that there are specific things you can do to decrease your pain.

## When and Why Does Pain Occur?

Pain is a message sent from your body to your brain saying that something is wrong. This painful signal begins when tissue is damaged or hurt. An electrical impulse is sent through the spinal cord to the sensory center of the brain, called the thalamus. The signal then goes to the brain's cortex or outer layer. Once the message is received in the cortex, you're able to determine the location of the pain and its intensity. Signals are then sent from the brain back through the spinal cord, triggering the release of natural painkillers such as endorphins—the body's own "morphine." This often diminishes the pain.

Although pain may initially be physical, your emotions can quickly worsen any pain you perceive. Anxiety or boredom, for example, can cause pain to appear more pronounced. Stress can cause muscles to tense, also increasing the degree of pain. Depression, too, may cause you to feel more pain, as it increases the tendency to focus on this sensation. And, of course, any pain you feel may increase the degree to which you experience anxiety, stress, or depression, which, in turn, can lead to more pain, creating a vicious cycle.

Other factors, too, may exacerbate the pain. For instance, fatigue may worsen pain by preventing your tissues from getting the rest they need to repair themselves. Your perception of pain may also vary based on your own tolerance, as well as the degree to which you think the pain can be controlled. So, you see, the experience of pain is highly subjective and affected by many factors. You'll want to try to control some or all of these factors in order to manage your pain more successfully.

What can you do about your discomfort? How can you cope with it? The best way to cope with pain is to get rid of it! To see if you can do this, it's first necessary to identify the cause of the pain. Once this is done, treatment can be aimed at eliminating the cause. But there's a problem. In some cases, it may be impossible to do anything about the underlying source of the pain. So pain itself, rather than the cause of the pain, is the most important concern. What does treatment aim to accomplish then? Relief from pain!

## Treatment for Pain

How can you start to deal with pain? First, you need to be aware of the pain. Keep track of when the pain occurs, how often it occurs, how long it lasts, and how intense it is. This will help you decide if the pain is something you can handle yourself, or if it's serious enough to be brought to your doctor's attention. Together you can work out the best way of dealing with it.

Despite the effectiveness of the pain control techniques mentioned in this chapter, it's important to consult your treatment team to determine which techniques are appropriate for you. Make sure that any techniques that you're thinking of using will not be dangerous for you, considering your condition.

Three general categories of treatment are used in the control of diabetes-related pain: medical treatment, physical therapy, and psychological strategies. All three types of treatments work by interrupting the transmission of pain messages before the brain receives and interprets them. Let's see how these three approaches can help you to control—or, ideally, eliminate—pain.

## MEDICAL TREATMENT

Medication may be used to provide relief from diabetes-related pain. In the case of mild pain, anti-inflammatory drugs may prove helpful. For example, two of the simplest nonnarcotic pain relievers are aspirin (acetylsalicylic acid) and Tylenol (acetaminophen). Nonsteroidal anti-inflammatory drugs (NSAIDs), another type of nonnarcotic analgesic, as well as narcotic pain relievers, can help to reduce pain. But sometimes discomfort will continue, despite the use of medication. And pain medication is generally not used for painful neuropathies. In extreme cases, surgery may be helpful in treating the cause of the pain. But very few cases really lend themselves to surgical treatment. So it may be necessary for you to learn other techniques for dealing with pain.

## PHYSICAL THERAPY

Transcutaneous electrical nerve stimulation (TENS) eases pain by blocking the transmission of pain messages to the brain. The TENS unit is a small box that contains a generator with anywhere from two to forty electrode wire leads. The electrodes are placed on the skin, on or near the painful area. When the unit is switched on, a low level of electricity flows into the area and stimulates the nerve fibers, thus blocking pain.

One problem with TENS is that its effectiveness seems to decrease over time. The effectiveness of this type of therapy is also dependent on your diligence, the knowledge of your therapist, and the placement of the electrodes.

Cold treatment may be beneficial in the temporary relief of discomfort, although it won't have an effect on diabetes itself. Cold has a numbing effect on nerve endings in the affected areas. It also decreases the activity of the body cells. (However, because of the importance of good blood circulation for people with diabetes, especially in the extremities, make sure your treatment team approves the use of cold for your pain.)

Gel packs, which can be obtained from pharmacies and medical supply stores, are an excellent means of applying cold, and because of their pliable consistency are often more comfortable than ice packs. These gel packs are kept in the freezer, removed for use, and then refrozen. Of course, if you don't have a gel pack, ice cubes placed in a plastic bag can be just as effective. But be sure to wrap either of these applications in a towel before holding it against skin.

## PSYCHOLOGICAL STRATEGIES

As we discussed earlier in the chapter, there are many factors that may influence your experience of pain, including anxiety, depression, and stress. Once you learn to control these factors, you're sure to feel a lot better. This is not to say that the pain is "all in your head." But pain is usually a combination of physiological and psychological factors. So although you may be experiencing true physiological pain, your mind is very much involved in determining exactly how much it hurts.

Carol was moving exceptionally gingerly, primarily because of painful neuropathy in her feet. The pain overwhelmed her every time she tried to step down. Even when she was doing something she enjoyed, her movements were restricted. Suddenly, she heard her five-year-old daughter begin to cry. Without thinking about her pain, she hurried across the room to comfort her daughter. So is Carol's pain all in her head? No. Sure, she had been in pain (and it was real), but when she had realized that her daughter needed her, the pain temporarily took on secondary importance.

What does all this mean? If medication and various physical therapies don't alleviate your pain, you can still relieve some—if not all—of it by working on your mind's perception of the pain. Many people have found effective pain control through the use of relaxation techniques, imagery, hypnosis, and biofeedback. These techniques work by separating you from your sensations of pain, enabling you to feel better. Some of these techniques may be learned at home. Others must be taught by professionals.

The following discussions should help you decide which of the psychological pain-control techniques may best help you as you learn to cope with diabetes.

## *Relaxation Techniques*

As discussed earlier, tension can actually increase your pain. So it makes sense that relaxation—the opposite of tension—can help you reduce your overall level of pain. As an added benefit, relaxation techniques may increase your general sense of well-being and help you to better deal with many day-to-day problems—not just those related to diabetes.

*Progressive relaxation* is based on the premise that when you experience anything stressful, the body responds with muscle tension—which, of course, can increase pain. In this procedure, which is usually performed for fifteen to twenty minutes once or twice daily, you sequentially tense and then relax the different muscle groups in your body, one group at a time. Most likely, you're already familiar with this popular and effective technique.

*Meditation* can allow you to achieve a deep level of relaxation in a short period of time. During meditation, you focus your mind, uncritically, on one object, sound, activity, or experience, and "clear out" any extraneous thoughts. Depending on the type of meditation you choose, this technique usually works best when taught by a professional or learned from a reliable book.

*Autogenics* is a systematic program that helps you train your body and mind to respond to your own verbal commands to relax. With this procedure, which can be used for short periods of time and repeated as frequently as needed, you give yourself verbal suggestions of heaviness, warmth, and calmness. Again, a book on relaxation techniques or a qualified professional can guide you in the use of this procedure.

Many people find that *deep breathing* can significantly increase their relaxation, and as a result decrease their pain. Deep breathing can be used in a number of different ways. Let's try a simple deep-breathing exercise together. First, assume a comfortable position on your bed or on the floor. Then put one hand on your abdomen and the other on your chest. Inhale slowly and deeply through your nose, so that the hand on your abdomen moves higher. Hold your breath as long as you're comfortable doing so; then exhale slowly through your mouth, making a peaceful "whooshing" sound. Feel the hand on your abdomen sink slowly, and allow a growing feeling of relaxation to deepen inside you. Repeat this sequence for five to ten minutes. Then give yourself a few minutes to become aware of your surroundings before getting up. Practice this technique at least twice a day, extending its length if you wish.

Another simple but effective relaxation technique is the *quick release.* Again, let's try this together. Close your eyes, take a deep breath, and hold it as you tighten the muscles in every part of your body you can think of—fists, arms, legs, stomach, neck, buttocks, etc. Continue to hold your breath and to keep your muscles tense for about six seconds. Then let your breath out in a "whoosh," and allow the tension to drain out of your muscles. Let your body go limp. Keep your eyes closed, and breathe rhythmically and comfortably for about twenty seconds. Repeat this tension-relaxation cycle three times. By the end of the third repetition, you'll probably feel a lot more relaxed. Keep on practicing this technique, as continuous practice will condition your body to respond quickly and completely.

Many other relaxation techniques may also prove helpful. Remember that your ability to increase relaxation and decrease pain by means of the mind-body connection is limited only by your imagination. Don't overlook this valuable way of improving your well-being.

## *Imagery*

Much research has indicated that bodily functions previously thought to be totally beyond conscious control can be modified using psychological techniques. Imagery, a technique that has grown in popularity over the last few years, uses this mind-body connection to help you cope with disease.

Imagery is the process of conjuring up mental pictures or scenes in order to harness your body's energy. In practice, imagery has been beneficial in helping people deal with a host of physiological and psychological problems. In addition to reducing stress, imagery has been successful in the control of headaches, hypertension, depression, and pain. Sometimes used alone, imagery can also be combined with prescribed medical treatment.

How can you use imagery to control your pain? Get into a relaxed position in a comfortable chair or bed. The lights should be dimmed, and outside sounds or noises should be minimized. Try to avoid interruptions. Breathe smoothly and rhythmically, allowing your body to release tension and relax. Then imagine a scene of your own choosing, trying to make the image as vivid and real as possible. This scene can be used therapeutically to help you feel better.

Ted was suffering from sharp pains in his feet. He was instructed to relax and then develop an image of what this pain looked like. He imagined it as dozens of very sharp pins sticking into his feet. Ted was then instructed to slowly reverse the action he had pictured. So he imagined the pins slowly being removed from his feet and a soothing, healing cream being applied. Ted was able to deepen his relaxation, greatly reducing his discomfort.

There are other images you can use to reduce pain. For example, you might imagine oil or a soothing lotion being gently massaged into the uncomfortable area, or you could picture yourself taking a warm bath. Imagery is restricted only by your creativity, and can be used anywhere. Two good books on the subject are *In the Mind's Eye* by Arnold Lazarus and *Visualization for Change* by Patrick Fanning. See if your local library or bookstore has them.

### *Hypnosis*

Hypnosis involves a calm repetition of words and statements designed to induce a state of deep relaxation in which there is a heightened receptivity to suggestion. During this state, verbal suggestions help the mind to block the awareness of pain and replace it with a more positive feeling. While hypnosis is often quite effective in the area of pain control, it doesn't work for everybody. Also, in some cases, it may not be as effective in dealing with severe pain.

You can learn how to hypnotize yourself so that you can use this technique whenever you need it. However, the technique must first be learned from a professional—a licensed psychologist, social worker, or certified hypnotherapist, for instance. Many good books on clinical hypnosis can give you further information about this valuable tool.

## *Biofeedback*

Biofeedback combines the techniques of relaxation and imagery, already discussed, with the use of electronic measuring instruments. These machines give you feedback in the form of sounds or images, letting you know what's going on inside your body. Biofeedback provides moment-by-moment information about the effect that your imagery and relaxation techniques are having on your physiological responses. What responses can be measured? Most frequently, the biofeedback units measure skin temperature, pulse, blood pressure, the electrical activity resulting from muscular tension, or the electrical activity coming from the brain.

How, exactly, can biofeedback help you control pain? Electrodes connected to the biofeedback unit are taped or otherwise attached to your skin. These electrodes monitor one or more of the physiological responses mentioned above, and transmit the information they pick up to the biofeedback unit in the form of electrical impulses. The unit then translates this feedback into sounds, lights, or pictures. Using this information, you can experiment and find the types of imagery and other relaxation techniques that will allow you to best control your internal responses, and thus induce relaxation and reduce muscular pain.

Glenda was experiencing a lot of neuropathy pain, so her physician suggested that she try biofeedback. As Glenda attempted to relax, the machine let her know if she was really relaxing and also how well she was relaxing. As she became more aware of her lessening tension, Glenda learned which mental images worked best for her. Eventually, she was able to use imagery on her own, without the machine, to help control her pain.

Check with your physician or local hospital or clinic for names of certified biofeedback professionals in your area.

## *Psychological Coping Strategies*

By now you probably understand the connection between emotions and pain, and want to do everything you can to decrease your fear, stress, tension, and other negative emotions—emotions that may make you more aware of pain or even increase it. Chapters 18 through 25 should help you pinpoint the source of your emotional distress, and then find ways of better coping with your feelings. Never underestimate the effect that emotions can have on your physical health!

Of course, the more time you have to think about your pain, the worse it will seem. So try to divert your attention. Develop interests that require concentration. You can always come up with activities that will entertain your mind while increasing your feeling of physical well-being.

## A Painless Conclusion

You can learn how to employ techniques for controlling pain from physicians, physical therapists, occupational therapists, and mental health professionals (such as psychologists who may specialize in certain pain control techniques). Or you may want to read some of the many books on pain that can be found in bookstores and libraries. Three good ones are *Free Yourself from Pain* by David Bresler, *Life Without Pain* by Richard Linchitz, and *Control Your Pain!: 169 Painless Strategies for Taking Control of Your Body* by Robert H. Phillips, Ph.D.

CHAPTER SIXTEEN

# Keeping Up with Your Activities

What to do, what to do? Sure, you have diabetes, but what does this mean in terms of the basic activities in your life? What can you do, and what can't you do? Each person is different. The kinds of things you did before being diagnosed with diabetes will influence what you can or want to do now. Your current physical condition is also an important factor. For example, if you have developed a diabetes-related complication, you may not want to expend a lot of energy until your doctor has given you the green light—or even a cautious yellow—to resume. So let's discuss some of the activities that may concern you, and see how you can make various kinds of changes that will enable you to be as active as you want to be.

## Working

Work helps you feel independent. It gives you a sense of fulfillment and self-worth. It provides more financial strength than not working, of course. And it is an important component of your social life. Understandably, you are probably quite concerned that your diabetes may interfere with your work. Perhaps you feel too tired to shoulder your usual workload. Let's look at some specific job-related concerns, and learn a little bit more about the ways in which diabetes can affect your work, and what you can do about it.

## SHOULD YOU CONTINUE WORKING?

Five basic points may help you when you are thinking about working. First of all, ask yourself if you feel comfortable doing the job. Do you feel physically and emotionally capable? Is it something you want to do? Your condition may have made you more determined to start doing something you really want to do! Second, does your employer still want you to work there? Or will a new employer hire you, given your present physical condition? Should you even say anything about it? (More about this later.) A third very important matter is whether your colleagues will accept you. This, of course, does not necessarily mean that they will even notice your condition. Fourth, will your condition and its treatment responsibilities affect your performance, attendance, or punctuality at work? If so, will this cause any difficulties on the job? A fifth factor that may relate to your choice of employment is the amount of stress involved. Becaue of the negative impact stress can have on your blood sugar level—not to mention overall health!—stress is certainly something you'll want to minimize.

## WHAT IF FATIGUE OR OTHER DISCOMFORTS ARE A PROBLEM?

You may be concerned that symptoms or side effects will prevent you from adequately performing on the job. Certainly, diabetes may cause you to experience fatigue and other discomforts, and this may affect your productivity—especially if your blood sugar is too high or too low. You may get tired easily, and feel that you just don't have the stamina necessary to complete your job satisfactorily. Your work rate may have slowed down, and you may be absent or late more than usual. If your employer is aware of any of these problems, you may be afraid that your value to the company will be questioned—that your job may be in jeopardy.

What should you do? Pace yourself. Take rest breaks whenever necessary—and possible—to "recharge your batteries." Build your stamina slowly. Don't expect too much all at once. If you're not sure how much you can do, do what you can and let your body be your guide.

Will your employer make any special provisions for you because you have diabetes? You may be able to continue working at a particular job with only a few modifications. For the most part, if your employer is satisfied with the work you're doing, there should not be a problem. But remember: You still have to do what you're supposed to do.

Of course, you may be uncomfortable about approaching your employer to find out if these changes can be made. It may bother you to seek "special treatment." But consider that any necessary modifications may be small in comparison to the ones your company would face if they had to hire a new employee to replace you!

What if your employer refuses to bend the rules? What if an ultimatum is given, stating that if productivity does not improve, you will be discharged? If this happens, simply do the best you can. If your employer doesn't understand enough about diabetes to know that you must pace yourself, and shows little or no willingness to cooperate, then you're probably better off not continuing employment there. You don't want to look for trouble.

What if another employee resents any special treatment you've been given? Find time to sit down, one-on-one, and have a conversation with your unhappy colleague. Explain your situation as much as necessary. Often, this is all that's needed to bring about greater understanding and cooperation. If your coworker still doesn't understand, content yourself with knowing that you tried. It's not your problem anymore. (For more information on dealing with colleagues, see chapter 28.)

## SHOULD YOU DISCUSS YOUR CONDITION WITH YOUR EMPLOYER?

How appropriate is it to discuss your medical condition with your employer? Well, some employers will be very supportive and understanding, while others will be somewhat apprehensive about retaining—or hiring—an individual who has any kind of physical problem. Use your discretion as to if and when you choose to discuss your diabetes with your employer . . . and how. Remember that your employer's primary responsibility is to keep productivity at its highest possible level. So it may be helpful to reassure your employer that you'll work to keep your condition from interfering with your own productivity. If, at some point, modifications do have to be made, you'll deal with them—and your employer—at that time.

## WHAT IF EMPLOYERS REFUSE TO RETAIN OR HIRE YOU?

If you are applying for a job, it's important to know which questions your interviewer is legally allowed to ask, and which questions must not be asked. For example, a potential employer can ask if you have any health or medical problem that would interfere with your ability to do the work involved in the position for which you're applying. Keep in mind, however, that this question cannot be asked in more general terms—an interviewer cannot ask whether you have a health problem. Also, by law, an interviewer is not permitted to list a series of medical problems and ask you if you have any of them.

It is not recommended that you lie about your condition during an interview. However, you can be circumspect about how much information you provide, and respond with only the bare minimum necessary. The best way to prepare for an interview is to rehearse. Ask a close friend or family member to bombard you with difficult questions. Practice your answers so that you can confidently and smoothly respond to these kinds of questions during your interview.

Once you have begun work, your employer can ask medical questions only with the intent to find reasons why you aren't able to handle the responsibilities of your position. Be aware that your employer is required by law to accommodate your special needs (within reason, of course). For example, your employer should allow you to adjust your work schedule so that you will be able to check your blood glucose, take insulin (if necessary), and eat snacks or meals according to your diet plan.

Employers may be hesitant to retain or hire someone with diabetes for a number of reasons. For instance, an employer may feel that health insurance premiums will be that much higher if you are listed on the plan.

But don't accept this argument. The Americans with Disabilities Act (ADA), most recently amended in 1997, clearly states that any employer with fifteen or more employees must not refuse you appropriate work or discriminate against you because of any disability. So if you are denied a job or dismissed from your present one because of diabetes, don't take it sitting down. Instead, call someone! For example, you can contact the Equal Employment Opportunity Commission (EEOC). Or check into resources such as your local bar association, which can direct you to an attorney who can help enforce the terms of the ADA.

## WHAT IF YOU HAVE TO CHANGE JOBS?

Because of new limitations, your old job may no longer be right for you. If this is the case, you should certainly consider transferring to another job, even if it means getting additional training.

Lenny, a forty-three-year-old father of two, was a successful public relations expert. But Lenny's doctors felt that he shouldn't continue doing this type of work, because of the high stress level and the number of times a week he had to wine and dine his clients. Lenny became very depressed. He didn't know what else he could do. Rather than face the prospect of being unable to work, he shut down emotionally.

Certainly the prospect of having to look for work is more daunting to some than it is to others. But if you are unable to continue working at your present job, don't despair. There are many ways in which you can get the training you need to move into a different type of position. Your first step might be to check with any of the government services that offer vocational counseling. Counselors in these offices will work with you to determine exactly what your aptitude is for different jobs. You will then be able to get the training and support you need to obtain employment in the desired field. If you need help finding jobs that are appropriate for you, your State Employment Services may be a good place to start. These services are available free of charge, and may guide you in locating jobs that will match your abilities and limitations.

Some people feel that for financial reasons you should postpone looking for new employment until your old employment has been terminated. This tactic has its pros and cons. If you receive unemployment benefits for losing your job, this could ease your financial burden. But if subsequent employers are reluctant to hire you because of your grounds for dismissal, this tactic may explode in your face. Only you, with your unique knowledge of your own situation, can decide which course of action is best.

### IS WORKING YOUR ONLY OPTION?

As you know, there are many benefits to working, including satisfaction, pride, and money. But a paying job is not the only type of satisfying work that's available. Many meaningful, productive activities can be pursued on a voluntary basis. Check with nonprofit charities, religious organizations, political groups, hospitals, schools, senior citizen centers, and the like. These types of organizations can always use some extra help. Volunteer work may even allow you to explore an area of interest that you've never been able to participate in before due to work commitments. And this work will help you feel good about yourself in the bargain.

What if you just don't want to work? If this is your preference, and you're able to manage without a job, that's great. But don't use your condition as an excuse for not working. Instead, try to find out what's really bothering you, and explore ways of eliminating the problem.

## Recreation

As we've mentioned in earlier chapters, it's vital to continue involving yourself in the activities you've always enjoyed. Why? Depending on their nature, of course, these activities may help keep you limber and vigorous. Just as important, they will provide a welcome diversion from any worries, prevent boredom and depression, and, very likely, put you in contact with other people.

Fortunately, most people with diabetes are able to participate in their normal recreational activities, including boating, skating, golf, tennis, dancing—the list goes on and on. What you do or don't do will depend solely on your own condition and, of course, on the recommendations of your health-care team.

## Activities of Daily Living

Among the things you do each day are numerous routine tasks—the activities of daily living (ADL). Of course, any restrictions you're experiencing because of diabetes may now be limiting these activities. If so, you're probably experiencing a lot of frustration. Why? Because prior to your diagnosis, you most likely took the accomplishment of these simple tasks for granted. And the way you're feeling now, you may be just too tired, depressed, or upset to look for a creative solution to these day-to-day problems.

What should you do? Well, you may not want to ask for help. You may feel that it takes away from your dignity. So you're stuck, right? Absolutely not! In a very short period of time, you can reorganize your lifestyle, your house, and your ADL in a way that will lessen your difficulties and salvage a lot of your dignity. How? Read on!

### SIMPLIFY YOUR TASKS

When learning to cope with ADL, keep in mind that your goal is to make daily living as easy as possible in order to conserve energy. You'll want to reduce or eliminate those activities that aren't necessary, and simplify those that are. This will allow you to avoid unnecessary fatigue, giving you the energy you need for the things you need—or want—to do.

How can you start? Well, begin by evaluating everything you do on a day-to-day basis. Then see how you can make every single thing you do easier. Is this taking the lazy way out? Of course not! You're simply recognizing that every bit of energy you save in the performance of one activity will give you more energy with which to do something else.

There are lots of things you can do to help yourself with daily living. For example, you can reorganize your home to make movement easier, and put the things you need within easy reach. Also, you might want to try wearing clothing that's easy to put on and take off—especially if you often have to spend a lot of time fiddling with buttons or zippers.

### PLAN AND ORGANIZE YOUR ACTIVITIES

In addition to eliminating unnecessary activities and making the remaining tasks easier to accomplish, you'll want to learn how to use planning and pacing to conserve energy. Try charting your activities, including your required tasks and your optional social and leisure activities. This may help you better organize your time. The more advanced the planning, the better—especially when big projects are involved—as this will give you time to figure out exactly how you're going to perform a given task, what equipment you'll need, and how the task might be broken up, if necessary, to allow for rest periods. Your local library and bookstores should have some excellent books on time management. Many of the tips in these books make such good sense that you'll probably wonder why you didn't think of them yourself! And every bit of time you save will be a big plus.

## A Final Exertion

By now, you've learned a lot about coping with diabetes, and you know that staying active is just as important as any other coping strategy. You want to feel productive and enjoy life. You don't want to let diabetes confine you to your bed or chair. Certainly you should modify any activities that are causing you discomfort, and you should do only what you physically can do—but *do* . . . !

CHAPTER SEVENTEEN

# Finding Financial Solutions

Having diabetes can be a pain in the pocketbook! Why? First, the bills for doctor's visits, laboratory tests, medication, supplies, and physical or occupational therapy all add up. Lost earnings, too, may add to costs if, for instance, you miss workdays because of diabetes. Certainly, the cost for each person—as well as the sources of these costs—varies considerably. But it may not take long for financial security to turn into financial troubles.

It is estimated that 15 percent of all health-care costs in the United States are connected with diabetes care and treatment for diabetes-related complications. This amounts to over $100 billion per year! Some estimates are that people with type 1 diabetes may have to spend as much as $4,000 per year. But before you begin to panic, you should know that you can reduce your costs. For starters, just by taking care of yourself and following your treatment as diligently as possible, you will help to control costs. What else can you do? Let's take a look at the many ways in which you can prevent or ease financial problems as you cope with diabetes.

## Talk to Others

If mounting medical costs threaten to engulf you, perhaps the first thing you should do is speak to other people. Through a support group, for instance, you may meet others in similar situations. Find out what they have done to control and meet the costs of their own care. Even though you may initially be embarrassed to bring up this subject, the common bond that exists among people with medically induced financial problems should quickly put you at ease. You'll be glad you brought it up!

For more ideas, you might contact your physician or another member of your health-care team. Make sure you express your financial concerns at the outset. This way, your health-care team can keep your financial needs in mind when they recommend treatment.

## Lower Medication Costs

If your treatment includes medications, the use of generic drugs may save you money. Generic medication is sold by its chemical name rather than the more common brand name, and is usually less expensive than the brand-name product. However, generics do not always work as well as their brand-name counterparts. Ask your physician if it would be acceptable to take the generic versions of any drugs you're currently using.

Some people try to cut costs by ordering their medications through the mail. This can be a legitimate way to save some money—but only if you deal with a reputable mail-order supplier. It's important to discuss this option with your doctor before you make *any* purchases. Ask your doctor and other members of your health-care team which companies—if any—they recommend.

## Attend a Clinic

If medical costs are overwhelming you, consider attending a clinic. Because clinics usually operate on a sliding-scale fee schedule, you may be able to receive quality medical care and equipment at a reduced cost. In some cases, you may even be able to continue seeing the physician who's treating you now; many physicians donate their time to clinics.

How can you locate a good clinic in your area? Your local hospital or your physician should be able to guide you to a local clinic that has the resources you need.

## Insurance Can Be an Assurance

Health insurance is essential, and a good health insurance plan is even more valuable. Many people have at least some of their medical costs defrayed by insurance. However, you may not be reimbursed for certain aspects of living with diabetes. For example, some insurance carriers will cover the cost of diabetes education; other companies do not consider this to be a covered benefit. Your insurance carrier may or may not cover the cost of medication or treatment supplies, including syringes, test strips, glucose monitors, and insulin pumps.

Most insurance policies have a deductible—an amount of money that you must pay before the insurance coverage begins. In addition, a small percentage of all costs may have to be paid by you, with the insurance company picking up the rest of the tab.

### GETTING THE MOST FROM YOUR INSURANCE POLICY

If you have a health insurance policy, contact your agent as soon as possible and find out as much as you can about your policy. (The policy itself will provide this information, too, of course.) Ask your agent the amount of your deductible, how many hospital days are covered, and how much is paid per day; how much coverage you have for surgery and anesthesia, whether or not second opinions are covered, and what your maximum lifetime coverage is. Also, make sure you know all of the procedures necessary to file a claim.

How can you help ensure that the process of claim filing and reimbursement runs smoothly? If you are responsible for the payment of your insurance premiums, make sure you pay them on time. Don't allow your insurance policy to lapse. And be sure to keep track of paperwork. Every time you send in a claim, keep copies of the claim form and of any attached doctors' bills for your own files. These may prove invaluable if a problem arises when your claim is processed. If, in fact, you do not receive a reimbursement on a claim, follow up by phone or letter, and request an explanation of the denial. If no satisfactory response is received, contact the insurance commissioner of your state, requesting an investigation.

Also keep records of the amount your insurance company pays on each claim, as well as the amount you pay on each claim. Your own payments may prove to be deductible on your next income tax return.

### WHAT IF YOU HAVE NO HEALTH INSURANCE?

If you are not presently covered by health insurance, you'll want to immediately contact all your resources—your accountant, your lawyer, your financial adviser, and organizations such as the American Diabetes Association, for instance—to learn about available options. The more individuals you contact, the more likely it is that you'll find the information you need. Of course, if you are unable to get any insurance coverage and are also unable to cover your medical costs yourself, you will probably be able to obtain assistance from government programs.

## Government Programs May Help

Government insurance programs are an important source of financial support for many people. You may be covered (at least to some degree) by Social Security Disability Insurance, Medicaid, or Medicare. Each of these plans have their own specific criteria for eligibility, and the criteria are often complicated, so you'll probably need to work with a professional to see if you qualify.

Let's take a closer look at these three programs:

## SOCIAL SECURITY DISABILITY INSURANCE

Disability benefits were added to the Social Security Act in 1956. An individual is considered to be "disabled" if he or she is unable to do any substantial gainful work due to a physical or mental impairment; and if the physical or mental condition is expected to last, or has lasted, for at least twelve months, or is expected to result in death.

The Social Security Benefit Plan is funded by workers and their employers. You must have worked five out of the ten years prior to your disability in order to qualify. This requirement may be reduced to one and a half years if the individual becomes disabled before reaching thirty-one years of age.

Benefits are available from the Social Security Disability Plan if you fit into any of the following categories:

1. Individuals under the age of twenty-two who are disabled before that age and are still disabled.
2. Widows who are disabled.
3. Widowers who are disabled and also dependent.

Even if you meet eligibility criteria for disability insurance, there are other steps that must be taken before you can collect any money. You will have to provide the names and addresses of people involved in treating you, including the members of your health-care team. Additionally, you'll need to list hospitals and clinics where you receive treatment. The Social Security Administration will need to see copies of medical records substantiating the dates you were treated and the treatments prescribed. Then a Social Security team, which includes a physician, will evaluate this information. Sometimes, additional tests are required to support a claim.

Once you apply for Social Security benefits, you also become eligible for Supplemental Security Income, or SSI. Like the Social Security Disability Program, the Supplementary Security Income Program is run by the Social Security Administration. However, SSI comes from a general treasury fund, rather than from workers and their employers. SSI benefits are available to individuals sixty-five and over, the blind, and the disabled. The eligibility requirements for SSI include the same definitions of disability that are used for Social Security benefits.

## MEDICAID

Medicaid offers benefits to individuals who are unable to pay for health care. This public assistance program is administered on the state or local level. Who qualifies for Medicaid? Virtually any low-income individual who demonstrates need can receive these public welfare benefits. Benefits are provided automatically for low-income individuals who qualify for Supplemental Security Income. Individuals who are sixty-five and over and who are receiving Social Security may qualify for Medicaid, and so may individuals who are under sixty-five and who have met the Social Security requirements for disability.

Medicaid will cover virtually any medical expense, as long as the health professional treating you is a participating provider. Your health-care provider is then directly reimbursed by the state for the service provided to you. If you have any questions about qualifications, or about the benefits themselves, check with your local welfare office for further information.

## MEDICARE

Medicare, a federal health insurance program, provides coverage for Americans aged sixty-five and over, and for disabled people of any age. Anyone, any age, who qualifies for and receives Social Security disability insurance also qualifies for Medicare after having been approved for two years. The degree of coverage provided by Medicare varies widely, so it's vital for you to determine exactly what health services Medicare will cover in your case.

Medicare is divided into two parts. Part A provides for anyone who has reached age sixty-five or is disabled, and is eligible for Social Security benefits. It covers hospitalization costs, as well as inpatient services in a skilled nursing facility. Part B covers doctor's charges, outpatient services, and specified medical items and services not covered under Part A. Part B insurance requires you to pay a monthly premium and a significant copayment.

While Medicare does provide coverage for large costs, it will not cover everything. For example, insulin is not covered under Medicare. However, the program does provide reimbursement for a number of different aspects of diabetes treatment. Up to 80 percent of the cost of blood glucose meters, as well as the supplies used with the meter, are covered by Medicare. The program also provides for foot care for people with diabetes. On the other hand, regular eye exams are not covered—but Medicare does pay for laser treatment for diabetes-related visual problems.

To determine whether any of these programs are applicable to you, contact your local Social Security office. In addition, consult your physician, your local support groups, or your local chapter of the American Diabetes Association. These sources can provide you with valuable information that will assist you in determining which programs can help you. But beware—these programs are strict. You can appeal if your application or claim is rejected, but this can be very aggravating. Want some advice? Talk to people who have been through it. Fight for your rights—and for your dollars.

## $umming Up

Financial concerns can be a big worry, but despite high costs most people are able to find ways to pay for appropriate treatment. The earlier you start planning, and the more qualified professionals you consult, the greater the likelihood that medical costs will not become a major problem for you. You will then be able to concentrate on your most important goal: living successfully with diabetes.

# PART THREE

# Your Emotions

# CHAPTER EIGHTEEN

# Coping with Your Emotions—An Introduction

How do you feel about having diabetes? The diagnosis can have a tremendous emotional impact on you, your family, your friends, and everyone around you.

Each person's emotional responses to diabetes are different. Even your own reactions to the condition will vary from time to time. The more severe your reactions are, the more they will interfere with your ability to cope. Your emotions can be like a roller coaster. As a matter of fact, emotional ups and downs are very common. But one of the most important aspects of being able to cope with diabetes is the ability to control your emotions.

Your emotional reactions to diabetes may start even before treatment begins. Of course, how you react will depend partly on how suddenly your condition develops. But there are many other factors—often in combination—that influence your emotional reaction to living with diabetes.

## The Factors Shaping Your Emotional Reactions

A number of factors may play a role in determining how you react to diabetes. Keep in mind, though, that because there are so many factors, no one can predict just how a person will react at any given time. How did you handle problems before your condition was diagnosed? What was your general coping style? Were you calm or nervous? Were you persistent or did you give up easily? The way you've handled life's problems in general will suggest how well you will cope with diabetes and its treatment.

Your age will also have a bearing on how you respond emotionally. Your general physical health prior to the onset of diabetes, too, will play a role in determining your coping ability. What about your relationships? In many cases, your emotional reactions may reflect the responses of significant others in your life. For example, if family members or friends are anxious about your medical condition, this may have an impact on the way you feel.

## Emotional Problems

Are you angry that your life will change because of diabetes? Are you afraid that diabetes will seriously impact your health in the future? Are you anxious about learning to give yourself insulin shots? Are you afraid of not being able to cope? Do you become depressed when you compare your present life with the way things used to be?

Virtually everyone who is diagnosed with diabetes becomes angry, anxious, and depressed. Feeling this way doesn't mean that you are weak. Rather, it means you are normal! Because of the importance of coping with these and other emotions, a separate chapter has been devoted to each. But other than these specific emotional responses, what else might you be experiencing?

You may become disoriented, as if the things around you are unreal. One of the most frightening feelings is that you're not yourself, especially if you don't know why you're feeling this way. It can be reassuring to understand that this happens to many people from time to time. And it can go away.

How about mood swings? Do you ever experience these? To some extent, these ups and downs reflect fluctuations in your blood sugar level. For example, you may feel more nervous or irritable when you have low blood sugar. On the other hand, high blood sugar may cause you to feel fatigued or depressed. But this doesn't mean that how you feel is due strictly to how high or low your blood sugar level is.

Everyone experiences mood swings from time to time. It's not uncommon to have some problems adjusting emotionally during times of major life changes, such as adolescence, going to college, starting a first job, getting married, or going through a pregnancy. Studies do suggest, however, that people with diabetes may find it more difficult to adapt to these major life events. For people with diabetes, the diagnosis of diabetes and (for some) the diagnosis of diabetes-related complications are other emotionally-charged life-changing events.

## Managing Emotional Reactions

Because your emotions play such an important role in your life with diabetes, you'll certainly want to do the best possible job you can of controlling them. How? Let's discuss some of the more important ways in which you can manage your emotions.

### GET THE BEST MEDICAL CARE POSSIBLE

Make sure you're getting the best possible medical care. If you haven't already done so, you'll want to establish a good working relationship with the members of your diabetes-treatment team. This involves seeing a doctor who not only has expertise in treating diabetes and is informed of the most up-to-date research, but who is also understanding, available, and sympathetic to your emotional needs.

## LEARN ABOUT MEDICATIONS THAT CAN HELP YOU COPE

There may be times when your emotions may get too intense. In some of these cases, you may want to consider medications that can help you cope. A number of medications can be effective in dealing with depression, anxiety, anger, and many other emotional reactions to diabetes. Antianxiety medications can be helpful, as can mood elevators and antidepressants. If you feel that you might benefit from treatment of this type, be sure to discuss the possibility with your doctor.

## JOIN A SUPPORT GROUP

Support groups can be incredibly helpful, and are some of the best sources of support for people with diabetes. Groups provide a forum for the exchange of feelings and ideas. Perhaps most important, these groups will show you that you're not alone—and it's much easier to live with a difficult problem when you know that you're not alone. It's helpful to meet new people who know what you're going through because they've gone through it themselves.

Members of support groups all have a common goal: to learn how to live as best they can, and to do as much as they possibly can. You'll see how others handle problems, some of which may be the same as, or at least similar to, your own. Learning how other people cope can be a tremendous source of support, especially if you really want to cope better but are not always sure how to do it.

Support groups can also be wonderful for your family, giving spouses, partners, children, parents, and others a chance to get some support of their own. And since one of the best ways to be in control of your emotions is to have a supportive family behind you, you should most certainly encourage their participation.

There are many groups run by professional leaders or facilitators that can be helpful to those with diabetes. These groups are great places to share your feelings and gain valuable information and strategies in a constructive, therapeutically beneficial way. Any topics you'd like to talk about can be discussed. You may begin to share feelings more openly when you hear others talking about subjects you were previously reluctant to bring up yourself. As a result, a feeling of closeness—almost a family feeling—will develop.

Don't feel that you *must* be in a group. If you're uncomfortable with the idea, or you don't think it's necessary because you're involved in other support activities, that's okay. Just make sure that you're honest with yourself. Don't feel that you have to share your emotional reactions with others. It's not necessary to talk them out, despite the potential benefits. But do realize that these emotions need to be recognized and worked through. That's the only way to make progress.

There are many different types of support groups. Contact your local chapter of the American Diabetes Association or the Juvenile Diabetes Foundation for more information about support groups in your area. These organizations bring patients and families together, and provide lots of beneficial information about diabetes and its treatment. You may also want to contact sources such as local hospitals or clinics, local schools of psychology or social work, religious organizations or libraries.

Finally, the Internet is a great way to find information about many aspects of diabetes. Not only will you find helpful Web sites that are devoted exclusively to diabetes, you can also visit chat rooms where you can share your experiences with other people in similar situations.

## EXPLORE PROFESSIONAL COUNSELING

Professional counseling can help whenever some aspect of your life becomes overwhelming, your emotional problems become severe, or you want to prevent problems from getting worse. Certainly, any period of change can be made easier with the help of a support professional such as a psychiatrist, psychologist, social worker, psychiatric nurse, pastoral counselor, or another professional with the necessary credentials, compassion, and expertise.

Having somebody to talk to can be a big help. When speaking to your counselor, it may be one of the few times when you can be totally honest in releasing your feelings, and at the same time get feedback that can help you better deal with your feelings. Yes, it can be helpful to talk to family and friends and to other people in your situation. But none of these people can provide you with the kind of frank intervention you can get from a therapist who is familiar with the feelings that exist when diabetes enters you life.

## USE EFFECTIVE COPING STRATEGIES

There are a number of coping strategies you can use to better manage the emotions that may be troubling you as you deal with diabetes. Any of these strategies can help you feel more in control.

Make a conscious, constructive agreement with yourself. Tell yourself that you're going to set aside a little time each day to work on strengthening your emotional self and preparing yourself for the next day. During this special time, include activities such as relaxation, imagery, goal setting, or positive thinking to improve your attitude. By consciously devoting time to this, you will improve your overall emotional state and increase your feelings of control, because you're doing something to help yourself.

Let's discuss some of the best techniques you can use to improve the way you feel.

### *Develop a Positive Mental Attitude*

It is so important to have a positive mental attitude. Individuals with good mental attitudes are much better able to take control of their emotions. A negative mental attitude may exacerbate any emotional problems that may occur because of, or in addition to, diabetes. So your primary goal should be to do all you can to improve your attitude so that you can improve every other aspect of your life.

Concentrate on the good. Why waste valuable time and energy focusing on the bad? Many books offer suggestions that can help you generate a more positive attitude. Look into some of these. If you get just one good idea out of a three-hundred-page book, the effort will be worthwhile.

Improving your attitude is a very important part of getting the most out of your life. If you think positive thoughts, you'll feel better, regardless of what's going on around you. Isn't that worth the effort? Walk tall, hold your head high, and feel good about who you are.

## *Laugh a Little*

Laughter is one of the most effective coping strategies there is. Research has shown that chemicals called endorphins—our body's own natural painkillers—are released by the brain whenever we laugh. These endorphins can block pain and give us a feeling of well-being. Haven't you felt better and experienced a greater sense of well-being after having a good laugh? You can enhance the process of getting and staying better by developing your sense of humor and making laughter an important part of your treatment program.

Humor is a pleasurable and effective way to deal with emotions. Whether you're listening to someone else's joke, laughing at yourself, or telling your own funny story, humor can be a big help in troublesome situations. Although there isn't anything funny about having diabetes, it helps to look on the bright side and lighten up a bit.

Humor works in three ways. First of all, it reduces anxiety. Laughter is one of the best ways known to release tension. Second, laughter can distract you from those feelings or thoughts that are bothering you. When you're involved in something humorous, you often feel a lot better. Think back, for example, to a time when you were depressed or uncomfortable, and somebody asked if you had heard a certain joke. Initially, you may have been reluctant to hear it. But before long, you were probably totally absorbed in the joke, wondering what the punch line would be! The fact that humor can distract you also means that it can help you to see things from a different perspective. So you may be able to look at something more objectively, which can help you to handle it more effectively.

Finally, the ability to laugh at yourself is a helpful coping strategy. The degree to which this works, however, depends on what you're going through. It's just about impossible to laugh at yourself while you're initially going through a crisis. However, as you adjust to your condition, you will be better able to use humor as a coping strategy.

So make laughter-filled experiences a part of your everyday life. Watch funny shows on television. Borrow humorous videotapes. Read amusing books or magazines. Listen to comedy tapes. Read the comics. Any of these things will help you have fun and feel better. Not only can they give you a quick boost by helping you distance yourself from what may be troubling you, but they can also improve your overall mood and physical well-being.

### *Make Use of Relaxation Techniques*

Relaxation is the opposite of tension. Therefore, if you learn to relax, you'll be much less tense! But relaxation techniques by themselves will not totally control your emotions. So why use them? Because if you're feeling more relaxed, you'll be better able to identify those problems that are affecting you, and you'll be better able to figure out how to deal with them. So relaxation procedures can be an essential first step in coping with your emotions.

How can you relax? We're talking about clinical relaxation, now—not everyday activities like reading, gardening, listening to music, or sitting in front of the television with a cup of coffee! There are several different types of clinical relaxation procedures, including progressive relaxation, meditation, hypnosis, autogenics, deep breathing, and a technique called the quick release. (Refer to chapter 15 for specific techniques.)

Remember that if you have difficulty learning to relax on your own, there's nothing wrong with working with a professional who can help you learn these skills.

### *Pinpoint What's Bothering You*

Are you more comfortable now? Then you're ready to proceed to the next crucial step. In order to deal with anything that's upsetting you, you have to determine exactly what it is that's bothering you! Make a list of these things. Then go over what you've written. In reviewing your list, you'll see that just about every item can be placed in one of two categories. The first category contains the "modifiables"—the problems or emotions that you can do something about. The second category includes the "nonmodifiables"—the things you can't do anything about. Why separate them? Because different strategies should be used to deal with each of these two types of problems.

For the first category, you'll want to figure out what techniques you can use to improve the situation. As for the second category, you'll still be planning strategies, but of a different kind! Where do your emotions exist? In your mind, right? Therefore, your plan for this category is to work on the way you're thinking.

### *Work on Your Thinking*

How can you change the way that you think so that something will bother you less? The technique you choose should depend on the specific emotional reaction that's bothering you. For example, if you're afraid of something and you want to conquer this fear, a procedure called systematic desensitization may be helpful. We'll go into this later in chapter 21. Then again, if you're feeling guilty or angry about something, or if something is depressing you, it can be very helpful to learn how to change or "restructure" the way you're thinking. You'll learn about more techniques for this in chapters 20, 22, and 23.

How do you deal with uncertainty? One of the first things to do is to focus on living as a person who happens to have diabetes, rather than seeing yourself as a victim of the illness. Try to live life and enjoy it as much as possible. Concentrate on what you have, not on what you don't. Concentrate on what you can still do, not what you can no longer do. Those who are successful are the ones who live life one day at a time, making the most of each day.

Actually, any of the techniques discussed can be used to cope with just about any problem. It's simply a question of deciding what works best for you.

## Looking Toward the Future

If you are presently experiencing intense emotional reactions, have faith that these feelings will diminish, either due to the passage of time or because you're doing something to help yourself. You can expect to experience more emotional reactions during those times when your symptoms are more pronounced or when your blood sugar is not well controlled, so you'll probably experience a range of emotional reactions from time to time. But even when these feelings do occur, you should be able to point to so many positive things in your life that it may be easier to deal with these feelings. In this way, you'll be able to develop the positive mental attitude that you want to become an integral part of your life.

The purpose of the following seven chapters is to help you understand the different emotions you may be experiencing. You'll discover where these emotions come from and come to recognize that many other individuals have gone through exactly what you're going through now. In addition, a number of strategies will be presented to help you cope with these emotions more effectively. Remember that "practice makes better." Just reading about a method to control an emotion doesn't guarantee success. You have to keep on practicing. So don't be afraid, depressed, angry, or guilty. Instead, read on!

CHAPTER NINETEEN

# Coping with the Diagnosis

It's only natural to feel overwhelmed after learning that you have a condition such as diabetes. After all, there's no easy way to accept the fact that your life is going to change. Initially, your mind may be filled with questions about what diabetes is and what the possible complications may be. So how can you possibly begin to cope? Calm down, take a deep breath, and be comforted with the knowledge that there are many things you can do to control your diabetes.

## Initial Reactions

When first diagnosed, you may not be able to react at all, since it may not seem "real" to you. But some people go through a hard time from the very beginning. It can be shocking to be told that you have diabetes, especially if you don't have any noticeable symptoms.

Emotional reactions to diabetes are not always rational. As a matter of fact, in many cases, they are completely irrational. And as the full impact of the diagnosis sets in, you may experience a whole variety of feelings ranging from sadness and anxiety to anger and frustration. You may feel upset because you'll have to make some lifestyle changes. You may be fearful that you'll never adjust to living with diabetes. No one—not even you—can predict how you'll react to the diagnosis, because no two people react in exactly the same way.

Let's look in greater detail at some of the more common reactions to the diagnosis. Later on in the chapter, we'll look at how you can begin to cope with these emotions.

## DENIAL

As discussed earlier, it's not at all unusual to deny that a problem exists. Regardless of the symptoms you've been experiencing, hearing that you have diabetes may provoke denial. You may protest, "Oh, come on. It can't be true," or "I'm sure the problem will go away by itself." You may even use more explosive, angry language.

Denial is especially risky in the case of diabetes. People who deny that the problem exists will not take steps to treat the condition and, as you've already learned, poorly controlled diabetes can lead to any number of short- and long-term complications.

There are two main ways that people with diabetes may act out their denial. First, there is denial that part or all of the treatment program is necessary. If this is the case, the person might completely disregard all of the components of their diabetes management plan. Some people ignore certain aspects of treatment, but adhere to others—for example, taking medication but not eating properly.

Second, there is denial that symptoms may suggest a progression of the illness or the development of a diabetes-related complication. For instance, a person who is experiencing blurred vision may not report this symptom to his or her health-care team. This may be an attempt to delay the doctor's discovery of a more serious problem.

Did you ever ask yourself, "Why can't I go back to the way things used to be?" Do you ever wish you could wake up one morning and find out that this was all just a bad dream? This is very common, but also very counterproductive. The more you keep hoping the situation will go away, the slower your adjustment will be. Why? Because you're not really admitting to yourself that you've changed—perhaps permanently. Rather, you're trying to push it out of your mind, hoping that things will return to the way they were. Try to recognize that your condition does exist now, that it affects you, and that it will remain with you. Then aim your efforts in the *right* direction. Try to plan your activities and structure all of your thinking toward handling your situation as effectively as you can.

If you're reading this book, chances are that you're probably not denying your condition. But if you are denying, somewhere along the line you're going to have to start facing reality. Speak to professionals who know about diabetes, and have them explain it in further detail. Let them tell you about the treatments available for your condition. Read about diabetes. Or talk to others with diabetes and listen to what they went through when first diagnosed. You will find that many of their experiences parallel your own. You'll also find that many of them have learned to adjust—just as you'll eventually adjust!

## ANXIETY

Immediately after the diagnosis, a commonly experienced reaction is anxiety. You may think, "Oh, no, what's going to happen to me?" Or you may ask, "What is the treatment—and how will I handle it?" "Will I ever get better?" "Who will take care of me?" "Am I going to die?" You may believe your life will never be the same again, because it will now include diabetes.

Let's talk about this reaction. It's normal to be upset and afraid. You may suddenly be hit with the fact that you are mortal and vulnerable. You'll realize you may have this problem for the rest of your life. Physically, it's not uncommon to feel faint or dizzy, or to experience other stress reactions at the time of diagnosis. Because of the tremendous fears that can immediately follow diagnosis—of loss of health or loss of independence—it's not surprising that this time is one of turmoil. The path to recovery from this turmoil is rarely smooth. A whole other group of emotions, such as rage, anger, and depression, comes into play as well.

Family members and loved ones may have the same fears and ask the same questions. They, too, may feel anxious and helpless because they don't know what they can do for you. This can certainly make things worse—for them *and* for you.

### RELIEF

You may be surprised to hear that some people actually are *relieved* when they are diagnosed with diabetes. Why? Because they knew they had a problem but didn't know what it was. At least they now know what it is so that treatment can prevent or minimize complications.

If you were experiencing different symptoms and nothing seemed to help, then the diagnosis of diabetes may give you hope—hope that treatment will improve the way you're feeling. Maybe you were afraid to go to the doctor, for fear that you would be diagnosed with a fatal illness. Then you're probably relieved to find out that your condition can be managed, and that you're not going to die. Perhaps you thought that your symptoms were purely psychological. Or maybe your family members didn't believe that you were experiencing physical symptoms. Well then, isn't it good to learn that there's a reason why you've been feeling this way—that is isn't "all in your head"?

## How Can You Begin to Adjust?

You may have many questions immediately following your diagnosis. However, the most important question is one that only you can answer: "Will I give up living because of diabetes, or will I continue to live despite diabetes?" The following steps should start you on the road to living successfully with diabetes.

### TAKE CHARGE

You must take the reins and begin to help yourself. Sure, you can receive love and support from your family and friends, and obtain guidance and expertise from professionals. But that's never enough. You are the one who is going to have to come to grips with diabetes. At first, adjusting may be a difficult struggle that requires tremendous effort. You may go through a lot of emotional turmoil. But there is no other way out. You must face it.

When you are learning to cope with diabetes, it's important to have a sense of empowerment—to be in control of as many factors in your life as possible. Because of the important role you play in managing your diabetes, you have to power to regain control of your health and live your life to the fullest.

## ACCEPT SUPPORT

If you're having a hard time accepting the diagnosis of diabetes, don't feel as though you should have to go through this experience alone. Reach out to family and friends for their support. You may be looking for a shoulder to cry on, or you may need some help getting your chores done or running errands. Recognize that this period of emotional adjustment is temporary—you won't be dependent on others forever. As we discussed in the previous chapter, you may want to join a support group. This is a good way to meet people who are experiencing the same feelings, or to learn from people who have already been through this difficult time.

## LIVE ONE DAY AT A TIME

You may feel overwhelmed when you consider the amount of self-care that is necessary to manage your diabetes. Starting a diet and exercise program, learning how and when to check your blood sugar, mastering your diabetes medications, keeping up with doctor's appointments—there's so much to learn and do! Is it any wonder that you might feel uneasy about the prospect of living with diabetes, at least until you adjust to the idea?

The best way to prove to yourself that you can manage your diabetes is to take life one day at a time. In fact, try taking your life one *step* at a time. Look at the components of your treatment program as a number of small, achievable steps. The more you repeat these steps, the more easily they will be integrated into your regular routine. When you are able to focus on and then master the different aspects of diabetes management, you'll quickly become more confident in your abilities to take care of yourself.

## INFORMATION, PLEASE!

Many of your initial reactions were probably the result of not knowing enough about diabetes. So you'll want to learn as much as possible. Your physician should be helpful in suggesting ways of getting current information.

It's very easy to let your imagination run wild. Initially, you'll probably keep thinking about all the things that can possibly go wrong. You'll worry about every symptom. You may also become frightened about developing diabetes-related complications. So learn the facts about your condition. This is a great way to alleviate some of the anxiety caused by the diagnosis.

After reading general, consumer-oriented information, you might want to move on to more technical material. Ask your doctor or diabetes educator about anything you don't understand. And certainly ask questions about anything that frightens you! After all, medical writing merely states medical facts and statistics—it's not necessarily written to comfort people with diabetes. Don't forget this, or you may become unnecessarily alarmed!

It probably wasn't a lifelong goal of yours to become an expert on diabetes, but think about how much this information may help you. Doctors will respect your questions more. And you'll understand exactly what's going on in your body. These are just two of the many advantages that can come from reading about your condition.

Should you believe everything you read? Of course not! There's no shortage of miracle "cures" and alternative treatments for diabetes. If a claim seems too good to be true, check it out to be sure the source is indeed reputable. New procedures and treatments must undergo rigorous scientific study to be proven effective. If you can't find credible scientific evidence to back up a claim, then you would be wise to stick with your current program.

The American Diabetes Association and similar organizations are committed to providing current information about diabetes and promoting public awareness of the illness. Many of these institutions also sponsor forums, recruit guest speakers, and organize clubs and self-help classes. You can also check out the Internet for more information about diabetes. There are dozens of helpful—and reputable—Web sites devoted exclusively to educating the public about this disease.

## BEGIN FACING YOUR FEARS

Once you've accepted the fact that you have diabetes, you can start determining what changes you may have to make in your lifestyle. In addition, you'll want to try to control as many harmful emotions as you can.

The emotions stemming from the diagnosis of diabetes can be unpleasant. You may experience regret, sorrow, nostalgia, and anger, remembering the way life used to be. Many fears may come to mind, some of which can be overwhelming. Fears of incapacitation, of being handicapped, or of losing out on life are all very common. Begin facing them. They can and must be faced in order to move your adjustment along more smoothly.

## DON'T DEMAND PERFECTION

In their attempts to keep their blood sugar levels tightly controlled, some people begin to feel an intense desire to perfect their self-care skills. Be careful! This kind of obsession can be very damaging. Remember: There are many factors that affect your blood sugar levels, and not all of these are totally within your control. Good control is certainly within your reach, but perfection is simply not possible. If you spend your life in pursuit of this unachievable goal, you'll quickly become frustrated—and you'll soon discover that you haven't left much time in your schedule for the activities you truly enjoy. So just do the best you can.

## DEVELOP A POSITIVE RELATIONSHIP WITH YOUR DOCTOR

Obviously, you must work with health-care professionals you can trust and who have had experience working with people with diabetes. You have the right—in fact, the obligation—to learn as much as possible about the different treatments for diabetes. And you can start by asking questions of your health-care team. If your doctor (or another member of your treatment team) does not seem receptive to your questions, try to make him or her aware of how important these concerns are to you. If no progress is made, then you may have to reconsider this relationship.

## HELP YOUR FAMILY ADJUST

It is understandably difficult to adjust to the diagnosis of diabetes and to cope with the many different emotions you are experiencing. This adjustment becomes that much harder when the people close to you also have difficulty with their emotions—especially if their emotions are different from yours!

Of course, it's easy to understand why family members might have trouble dealing with the diagnosis. They, too, will go through periods of denial—times at which they'll say, "No, everything will be fine," or "I'm sure the problem will clear up by itself." Unfortunately, this won't make things easier for you.

Louise, a secretary, was thirty-nine years old when she was diagnosed with diabetes. After a couple of very depressing months, Louise started to learn how to cope. She was finally able to handle thoughts of lifestyle changes, concerns about restricted diet, and some of the other unpleasant realities associated with her condition. Sound great? Not really. You see, Louise's husband of fifteen years could not accept the fact that she had this problem, her children were afraid she was going to die, and her sixty-two-year-old mother was having a hard time dealing with guilt. Although Louise was learning how to cope with diabetes, she could not cope with her family.

It's a great idea for family members to seek out people to speak to—just as it may benefit *you* to seek help. Spouses, children, and others can find out more about diabetes and learn how others cope with treatment. They can even join support groups or seek counseling. So encourage your family and any willing friends to learn as much as they can and to seek whatever help they need. Their adjustment will help your adjustment.

## In Closing

Start thinking positively about your life with diabetes. Learn as much as you can about your condition. Use whatever support systems are necessary. Use all of the stress management and emotional control techniques you can learn. (Many good ones can be found in this book!) Start saying to yourself, "Diabetes may be a part of my life, but I'm still alive, and I'm going to do whatever I can to help myself adjust."

If it's necessary for you to make changes in your lifestyle, tell yourself that you will make them, and that you will learn to live with them! You're going to lead as complete a life as you can. The more quickly you can adapt your lifestyle to fit your needs, the more rapidly you'll be able to enjoy your life. This may be hard at first, and will certainly take time. But you're not helpless, and you can take steps to make the most of your life despite diabetes!

# CHAPTER TWENTY

# Depression

Stan was feeling very down. A fifty-eight-year-old father of three, married for thirty-four years and living in a beautiful home in a good neighborhood, he apparently had everything he could ask for. But he certainly hadn't asked for diabetes! He found himself feeling increasingly upset about the changes that had to be made in his life. He was afraid that he would have to restrict his activities because he needed insulin shots. He thought that "eating healthy" would mean he'd have to give up the foods he loved. Most of all, he worried about developing diabetes-related complications. He felt helpless and hopeless. In short, Stan was suffering from depression.

Depression is a serious problem. Although actual numbers vary, it is estimated that more than 5 million Americans need professional care for depression. Because it is so widespread, depression has been nicknamed the "common cold" of emotional problems.

Just what is depression? Depression is an extremely unpleasant feeling of unhappiness and despair. It can range from a mild problem—feeling discouraged and downhearted—to a severe disorder—feeling utterly hopeless, worthless, and unwilling to go on living. You may believe that there is no reason to remain a part of the world. You may be afraid of being a burden to your family, and think that everybody would be better off without you. Or you may just feel useless.

Depression can be painful. Imagine how it must hurt to feel (or say), "I wish I were never born. What good am I? I'm not helping anybody around me, and I'm not helping myself." You may feel as if the whole world is against you. Life may seem unfair—a constant struggle in which you can never win. And that hurts.

## What Are the Symptoms of Depression?

There are a number of possible symptoms of depression. If you notice that you're feeling excessive amounts of sadness, despair, discouragement, or melancholy, if you're unable to eat, and this problem has nothing to do with the diabetes or its treatment, if you're sleeping either too much or too little, if you feel totally withdrawn from social activities, if you find yourself crying often, and that's not typical behavior for you, if you're brooding about the past and feeling hopeless—any of these feelings may indicate depression. And there are other symptoms, as well. If you're experiencing excessive amounts of irritability or anger, if your fears seem to be extreme, if you feel inadequate and worthless, if you are unable to concentrate on virtually anything in your life, whether it be work, family, or other interests, if you seem to have little or no interest in activities that previously gave you pleasure, if you have reduced amounts of energy that don't seem to be related to the disease or treatment, if you have little or no interest in sex or intimacy, and if your cognitive style (the way you speak, think, and act) seems to be generally slowing down—these, too, can be symptomatic of depression. The more of these symptoms you experience, the more likely it is that you are depressed and should take some action to help yourself.

## How Does Depression Affect You?

Now that you are familiar with some of the many possible symptoms of depression, you should also be aware that its effects are not isolated problems. Depression can affect your physical well-being, take control of your moods, and make it difficult to enjoy—or even carry out—the simplest activities. Let's take a look at some of the ways in which depression can affect your day-to-day life.

## HOW DEPRESSION AFFECTS YOUR BODY

Some of the more noticeable symptoms of depression are physical in nature. Nervous activity or agitation, such as wringing of the hands, may occur. You may be restless or have difficulty remaining in one place. On the other hand, you may become much less active and remain motionless for abnormally long periods of time, appearing to be almost in a trance, with no desire or energy to do anything.

If you're depressed, most of your physical activities will also slow down—and not just because of physical limitations. You're probably feeling exhausted. This may be surprising, since you're not doing much of anything. But constantly telling yourself that you're no good can be tiring in itself! You really don't want to believe this, but you feel as if you have no choice. And in attempting to escape from these feelings, you may become even more depressed—as well as more physically drained and exhausted.

Depression may also cause you to feel physically sick, or to experience a change in appetite. Of course, it's wise to remember that any of these symptoms might be related to diabetes or another physical disorder. So even if the symptoms go away once your depression improves, don't just assume that they're related to the depression. A medical examination may still be a good idea. This way, you'll be sure that there is no organic cause for your depression.

## HOW DEPRESSION AFFECTS YOUR MOODS AND OUTLOOK

If you're depressed, you may experience frequent mood swings. For example, you might feel worse in the morning and better in the evening. This nightly improvement may occur because each evening you realize that it's almost time to go to sleep—to escape. But depression may also make sleep difficult, even if you weren't doing much of anything during the day. If you're mildly depressed, you may have difficulty concentrating, and your attention span may be much shorter. When you speak, your conversation may suggest, or even express, feelings of worthlessness and despair.

When you're depressed, it feels as if your mood keeps getting lower. You like yourself very little, if at all. Your thinking is very negative and very different from the way it was when you were feeling good. In fact, it is this negative thinking—not just a particular triggering event—that leads to depression in the first place. (But more on this later in the chapter.)

Naturally, your day-to-day activities may suffer as a result of these negative feelings. You may, for instance, spend the day in your bathrobe simply because you don't feel like dressing. Or you may "go through the motions" of your everyday activities, even though your heart isn't in them. Many people, in fact, simply withdraw from their usual activities during bouts of depression.

## HOW DEPRESSION AFFECTS YOUR RELATIONSHIPS WITH OTHERS

Do you now feel less at ease talking to others? Does it seem as if others are having a hard time talking to you, even if they have been close to you for a long time? As already discussed, due to your depression you may be less interested in conversation and you may feel less confident. You may project your negative feelings about yourself onto others, and believe that they really don't want to talk to you. And the more depressed you become, the better you may get at convincing those around you that you're no good. You may feel that others have no need for you. You may think that they consider you to be an uninteresting, boring person.

Anita received a telephone call from her friend Ruth. Ruth wanted to know how Anita had been feeling, since the last time they had gotten together Anita had seemed fatigued. Anita responded halfheartedly, imagining that Ruth was calling only out of obligation. She then explained that she would understand if Ruth did not want to call again, since she never seemed to have any good news to tell her. How do you think Ruth felt?

Imagine hearing this repeatedly! Would you be surprised if eventually Ruth got tired of even trying, and simply stopped calling? But in Anita's mind, this would only reinforce the fact that she really was no good—that she was not worthy of having any friends after all!

## What Causes Depression?

Where does depression come from, and why does it sometimes take hold? Sometimes we can figure this out, and sometimes we can't. But before we give up, let's discuss some of the possible causes.

### HOW ABOUT THE "NORMAL DOWNS"?

A certain amount of depression is normal in anyone's life. We all experience ups and downs. If we never experienced some of the downs, how could we ever fully appreciate the ups? However, when depression becomes more than just the "normal downs," it must be attended to. Nipping it quickly in the bud can keep it from becoming much worse.

Of course, certain events—traumatic experiences such as losing a loved one, being diagnosed with a chronic medical problem, requiring major surgery, or being fired from a job—can lead anyone to depression. However, this doesn't mean that you should ignore the problem or wait until it goes away. It's necessary to learn how to deal with depression, as this is an essential part of coping.

### HOW ABOUT ANGER YOU CAN'T EXPRESS?

What if you get so angry that you feel like you're going to burst? But you don't—or can't—do anything about it, so you decide to "swallow" your anger. It seems strange that a powerful feeling like anger can turn into a withdrawn, helpless feeling like depression. But it can. If you become increasingly angry about something and feel unable to do anything about it, you may turn the anger inward. You may feel so much frustration or hopelessness that you "shut down" in an attempt to keep yourself from experiencing these terrible feelings. This leads to withdrawal, which is one symptom of depression. (For more information on anger, see chapter 22.)

## DIABETES AS A CAUSE

Living with diabetes can certainly either create or magnify already existing depression. So it is not surprising that a certain degree of depression may occur after the diagnosis. Some research has suggested that depression is more common for people with diabetes than it is for people in the general population. It also seems to recur more frequently and may last longer.

One contributor to depression in people with diabetes may be the realization that some lifestyle changes will have to be made. For example, you may be depressed if you have to set aside time every day to check your blood sugar or give yourself insulin shots. Or you may feel unhappy because you need to watch what you eat a little more carefully. And it's only natural to feel depressed thinking about the future, wondering how diabetes will affect your life.

What else about diabetes may depress you? Problems involving other people may depress you. You may believe that others don't understand what you're going through, and this can cause you to feel down. People may expect more from you than you're able or willing to provide. You may be depressed over the possibility of damaged relationships, lost friendships, or family friction. But there need not be any truth to this at all!

You may be saying to yourself, "If I'm depressed about my diabetes, how can I expect to get over my depression unless my diabetes is cured?" That kind of thinking will get you nowhere. You can't ignore the fact that diabetes is a chronic condition—and you don't want your emotional state to depend on your physical state. So if your depression lingers, don't wait. Work on it, and learn how to cope. We'll talk more later about how you can improve your thinking.

## What Maintains Depression?

If you're depressed, you may be blaming yourself—or your diabetes—for everything that is wrong. You may tend to become more and more withdrawn, and pull away from the world around you. Why? Well, if you believe that your condition is causing all these horrible things, isn't it better to "escape" and not think about it? Realistically, escaping won't solve anything. But you may feel that withdrawal is the only way to stop feeling terrible. Unfortunately, this will only keep you depressed. (In fact, it may make you even more depressed.)

Although you may even seem sullen and withdrawn to others, you're probably in deep emotional pain. Part of what is making you, and keeping you, depressed is your effort to protect yourself from this emotional pain. When your mind does allow any thoughts to enter, you tend to be overwhelmed by feelings of doom and destruction. You feel that nothing good can possibly happen—that only bad things can happen. So what do you do? You try to block everything out of your mind!

So why do you stay depressed? Why doesn't it just go away? It may be because you don't want to talk to anybody, or even consider counseling. Therefore, the thoughts and feelings that lead to your depression are kept hidden. You may ask, "Is my unwillingness to talk the only reason I'm still depressed? If I start talking more, will that get me out of my depression?" Not necessarily. But it can be helpful to talk out your feelings. It would probably be beneficial if a close friend or family member took the initiative and forced you into some kind of conversation—therapeutic or otherwise—or at least pushed you into doing something constructive.

## How Can You Cope with Depression?

Can anything be done to end depression? Of course! Make sure that, in your efforts to help yourself feel better emotionally, you also concentrate on taking care of yourself physically. Remember that high blood sugar can exacerbate your depression; therefore, one of your first steps toward alleviating the depression should be to bring your blood sugar under tight control, if you have not already done so.

You next step will be to tell yourself that the main reason you're depressed is that you haven't taken the proper steps toward emotional wellness. These steps can pull you out of your rut and reacquaint you with the more positive, pleasant aspects of living—the aspects that you'd like to experience.

Don't think it will be easy, though. Unfortunately, once you've fallen into depression, it takes hard work and a certain amount of persistence to pull yourself back out. The result, however, is surely worth the fight. And, of course, the fight will be easier if you know of specific techniques and activities that will help. Don't be afraid of depression. Rather, expect it and prepare yourself for it. This will help you better deal with depression when it does occur.

The strategies and techniques that are most effective in dealing with depression can also be effective in preventing you from becoming depressed. Unfortunately, this doesn't mean that you'll never again feel depressed. It may happen. Anticipate it, so that if it does recur you won't completely fall apart. And if this feeling comes back, won't it be good to know that you *can* do something to help yourself?

Now that you're ready to fight your depression, consider two major ways of dealing with it: being more physical (in other words, doing something) and working on your thinking. It can be very helpful to make a list of all the things that are depressing you. You may feel there'll be at least fifty items! But in actuality, you'll probably start running out of ideas after six or seven. Next, divide this list into two more lists: first, those things that you can do something about, and, second, those things you can't do anything about. So get physical and do something about those items on the first list, and get thoughtful—work on your thinking—regarding those items in the second list.

## LET'S GET PHYSICAL

There are two ways of getting physical in order to deal with depression: actively working to accomplish goals, and increasing physical activity. Hopefully, as suggested on page 219, you've listed all the things that are depressing you, and have made a separate list of those items that can be changed. Now think about ways in which you can modify or eliminate the items on this list. Be realistic but aggressive in planning ways to reach your goals—even if they can't be done all at once.

Where does the physical activity come in? Unknowingly, you may be using a lot of energy to keep yourself depressed. You may be working hard to keep that anger inside, even if it appears to others that you're simply withdrawing. If your depression is anger turned inward, we can logically assume that by releasing your anger you'll be able to eliminate your feelings of depression. But what should you do with those feelings? You must find an object toward which your anger can be expressed. This may be difficult. However, it's important to release the trapped anger so that it doesn't build up further and deepen your depression.

Think about the following scenario. You're sitting there, depressed and withdrawn. Somebody makes an innocent remark, and you practically bite that person's head off! What's happening? Whatever was said triggered the release of the internalized anger that was making you depressed. Look out, world!

What kinds of activities can help you release your anger? Many physical activities can be effective. Exercise helps by lowering your blood sugar level, and it also causes the release of neurotransmitters called *endorphins.* Endorphins make people feel good and can give them a more positive attitude.

Before you begin any exercise program, you should schedule a complete physical to make sure that exercising is safe for you. Your physician or exercise specialist will help you develop an appropriate exercise regimen. If you have a diabetes-related complication, you can still choose an appropriate exercise program, but you need to make sure that physical activity will not contribute to further harm. It's very important that you're clear on which activities are safe for you, so you must work closely with your health-care team to plan a program that will provide maximum benefits with little or no risk. (Refer to chapter 9 for a complete discussion on setting up—and sticking with—an exercise program.)

## LET'S GET THOUGHTFUL

Although getting physical may help lift your depression—and can also provide a great distraction, which may help you to look more objectively at what's going on—physical activity will not teach you ways of fighting inappropriate thinking. Remember that it's your *thoughts* that have made you depressed. Clearly, restructuring you thinking is a key element in alleviating depression and dealing with any negative emotions.

If you can think yourself into depression, then you can think yourself out of it. How? If you're depressed, you're just talking yourself *down.* All your comments—or at least most of them—are probably put-downs: harsh statements that can make you feel even worse. You want your inner voice to help you, not hurt you. Let's see how you can do that.

### *Distinguish Fact from Fiction*

When you're depressed, you tend to distort reality. Clinical research with depressed patients has proven this. Recognize, therefore, that your thoughts are not necessarily based on what is really happening, but may instead be based on your own distorted views. This is called *cognitive distortion.*

Is this bad? You bet your happiness it is! *Cognitive* refers to your thinking. *Distortion* means you're twisting things around and in general losing sight of what's real. We all tend to do this from time to time. But when you're depressed, you do it a lot of the time—if not all of the time—and it keeps you depressed. So how do you stop? First, you must become reacquainted with what is really happening. But how can you do that if you keep distorting reality? Right now, you're better off accepting somebody else's perceptions of the situation, because that person is probably a lot more objective and accurate. Since so many feelings of worthlessness are based on distorted facts, depression can be reduced, if not eliminated, once these facts are straightened out.

Ellen kept moaning because none of her friends were calling her. "They don't call as much as they used to. I guess they just don't care." Her daughter, Laurie, asked her to estimate how often her friends used to call. When Ellen compared this number with the current number of calls she was receiving, she realized that the numbers were almost the same. She then recognized that she was probably just more sensitive because of all the changes going on in her life! Although she did not feel a hundred percent better, Ellen did feel a good deal better, because she could now see that she hadn't been abandoned.

So make sure you know what's true and what's not. Provide your own assessment of the situation, and be as objective as possible. Then, if necessary, ask other people—people whose opinions you trust—for their evaluation. Work to become more comfortable with any differences in perception and to adjust your thinking so that it more closely resembles the actual circumstances.

### *Making Molehills Out of Mountains*

Does this imply that if you're depressed you have no real problem? Is it "all in your head"? No. Everyone has problems. If you feel good, you can handle them; but if you're depressed, you may feel overwhelmed. Each and every obstacle and task, regardless of how trivial or slight it may be, will tend to depress you.

Again, do your best to view each problem objectively—to avoid blowing it out of proportion. Eventually, as your depression lifts, you will be able to deal with all of life's problems, both big and small.

### *Avoid Self-Fulfilling Prophecies*

We've discussed several thoughts that are characteristic of depression—thoughts that you may be having right now. Are all of these thoughts and feelings irrational and untrue? No. But ironically, although some of them may start off being far from the truth, the longer you feel this way, the greater the chance of their becoming self-fulfilling prophecies. In other words, the more you allow yourself to think negatively, the greater the likelihood that your fears will turn into realities. For example, if you begin telling yourself that friends and relatives don't care, this may become a reality, because your negative attitudes may alienate the people close to you. And if you feel less able or less willing to do the things you used to do, your inactivity is likely to magnify and confirm your feelings of worthlessness, leading to even greater depression and helplessness. Not a pretty picture.

Once you begin feeling depressed, your negative thoughts will soon lead to negative actions. These negative actions will lead to more negative thoughts, which will in turn lead to more negative actions, and so on. It is an ongoing, vicious cycle that will spiral you further downward into deeper depression. Eventually, you'll feel trapped in this vicious cycle, and believe there's no way to escape.

Are you getting depressed just reading this? In all probability, if you've ever been depressed you've said to yourself at least once already, "Wow, that sounds just like me!" So if you find that you're starting to believe your negative thoughts, stop yourself. As we've said before, depression both results from and causes a lot of negative thinking. But once you become aware of these thoughts, you can do something about them. People who remain depressed feel incapable of doing anything about their negative thinking, and allow these thoughts to pull them into that vicious cycle mentioned earlier. Try to think positive thoughts, so that if one of your thoughts does turn into a reality it will at least be a positive one.

### *Dwell on the Brighter Tomorrows*

If you find yourself unhappily comparing your present life to life before diabetes, try to modify your thinking. Start planning fun things for the present and future. Anyone can come up with some enjoyable activities, regardless of physical restrictions. But it takes effort. Don't wallow in self-pity, because that will only allow your depression to overwhelm you. Develop some positive plans, and translate them into pleasure. Then wave good-bye to your depression!

Of course, if you clearly reflect on your past, you may find that it wasn't much better than the present! In the past, you may have had other physical problems. You may have made some mistakes. Naturally, this may make you even more depressed about the future. However, you can't change the past. What's done is done. Keep telling yourself that. Don't punish yourself for the past. Tell yourself that you're going to work on making the future better. Set up some specific goals, starting with the easy-to-reach ones. You'll be helping yourself just by *thinking* about all the positive things you can do!

### *Rediscover What's Missing from Your Life*

You may have laughed when you read the title of this section. "Insulin!" you might respond. Sure. But another important element that might very well be missing—an element that can be regained!—is the feeling of satisfaction, accomplishment, and pride that normally comes from others' praise. You may be missing the attention and interest of other people, and this can cause you to feel worthless. What can you do about this? Think about your positive qualities. (Yes, you do have some!) Think about how you can interact more with people, spark their interest, and obtain more of the satisfaction that makes you feel worthwhile.

### *Shoot for the Earth, Not the Moon*

We all have goals for ourselves. It's normal to become depressed when we don't reach a particular one, especially if we've tried very hard to get there. But sometimes our goals are not realistic. Try to judge if the goals you've been setting for yourself are realistic. If not, reset them, keeping your abilities and limitations in mind. Once your goals are more realistic, you'll have a much better chance of achieving them, and less chance of falling short.

Bill had not returned to work since a recent hospitalization. Finally, after a period of rest and rehabilitation, he was feeling better. His diabetes was under control, and he was looking forward to getting back to work so that he could catch up on what he had missed. When his doctor finally gave him the go-ahead, he practically flew to his office . . . and after two hours of phone calls, consultations, dictation, and meetings, he was exhausted and his spirits plummeted. As a result, Bill became worried that he'd never again be able to handle all the pressure, when in reality he had simply set his sights too high. Expecting to return to his old schedule as if he hadn't been in the hospital was just not realistic. Instead, he should have taken more time to build up his stamina and ease his way back into his normal routine.

### TALK ABOUT IT!

Now you know how to cope with depression through both physical activity and by changing your way of thinking. But there's one more thing you can do—something discussed earlier. You can talk about your problems and concerns with others. Often, the very act of talking will help lift your depression. If there are family members or friends whom you feel close to and whose opinions you trust, talk to them. Air your feelings and listen to their feedback. They may be more objective, and better able to come up with constructive solutions.

If your depression is so intense or prolonged that friends and family are unable to help, then by all means consider speaking to a professional. Counseling is a very effective way to treat depression. So don't deny yourself this invaluable assistance. Why not do everything you can to help yourself feel better?

## When Are Antidepressants Appropriate?

In a small percentage of cases, depression may be caused by biochemical deficiencies—chemical imbalances in our bodies. If depression is persistent, and nonmedical coping strategies are not effective, then antidepressant medications may prove helpful. Examples include tricyclic antidepressants such as Tofranil (imipramine hydrochloride) and Norpramin (desipramine hydrochloride); and MAO (monoamine oxidase) inhibitors such as Nardil (phenelzine sulfate) and Parnate (tranylcypromine sulfate). These medications work in different ways, and result in different possible side effects. Other antidepressants include Desyrel (trazodone hydrochloride), Elavil (amitriptyline hydrochloride), Ludiomil (maprotiline hydrochloride), Pamelor (nortriptyline hydrochloride), Prozac (fluoxetine hydrochloride), Zoloft (sertraline hydrochloride), and Sinequan (doxepin hydrochloride).

There is always the chance that certain medications may not be appropriate in your diabetes treatment program. *Always* check with your doctor! Question, learn, and help yourself. If you need to take many different pills, it's important to avoid playing with your dosage and with the times you take them, or moving around the number of pills you take at a particular time. Follow your doctor's prescription as carefully as possible. In addition, be careful about bad mixes. Some mixes can make your symptoms worse, interfere with the action of the prescribed medication, or cause additional problems. Don't hesitate to ask questions.

Because medication causes chemical changes within the body, side effects may occur whenever a drug is taken. And, unfortunately, the more powerful the drug, the more potent its side effects may be. If the side effects you experience are slight, you will probably want to ignore them—especially if the medication you're taking is having the desired effect. If side effects are having a harsh impact on you, let your physician know, so the two of you can weigh the disadvantages of the medication against the advantages. In fact, any side effects should be reported to your doctor so that he or she can determine if the drug therapy should be continued, changed, or ended.

Regardless of whether your depression is caused by a biochemical deficiency or by your reaction to the people and events around you, you should still try to modify your thinking. Many experts believe that even if the cause of depression is biochemical, by working on the way you handle your day-to-day living you can have a positive effect on your emotions.

## An Antidepressing Summary

The best way to work on negative thoughts is to prevent them from continuing. Try to be realistically positive. Deal with reality the way it actually exists. Deal with thoughts from a more factual point of view. Handle them the way they might be handled by somebody else—somebody who is not depressed and who can be more objective. Try to make your perceptions more accurate, your awareness more realistic, and your thoughts more constructive. Remember: Your thoughts lead to your emotions. If your thoughts are negative and critical, your emotions will be the same. But if you can turn your thoughts around to a more positive, constructive point of view, your emotional reactions will most certainly follow. And depression will then be a thing of the past.

## CHAPTER TWENTY-ONE

# Fears and Anxieties

Don't be *afraid* to read this chapter! It may help you to discover what you're *anxious* about!

The two sentences above may help you to distinguish between anxiety and fear. What's the difference? Anxiety is a general sense of uneasiness—a vague feeling of discomfort. It is an agitated, uncertain state in which you just don't feel at peace or in control. There is a premonition that something bad may happen, something you have to protect yourself against. You feel very vulnerable. However, you're not exactly sure what the source of your anxiety is.

Fear, on the other hand, is usually more specific. It's often directed toward something that can be recognized, whether a person, object, situation, or event. We have fear when we become aware of something dangerous, or when we feel threatened. When we are afraid—much like when we're anxious—we feel out of control and less confident. So the feelings of anxiety and fear are basically the same, the main difference being whether the source of the feeling can be identified. For this reason, from this point on I'll be using the two terms interchangeably.

Fear is so common that we have developed a number of different words to describe it: scared, concerned, alarmed, worried, uptight, nervous, edgy, and shaky. Then there's wary, frightened, and helpless. Is that it?

Nope! How about suspicious, hesitant, apprehensive, tense, panicky, disturbed, and agitated? Of course there are more, but you get the general idea. The important point is that all these words mean the same thing: "I'm afraid." The source of this fear may be either real or imaginary.

## What Are the Symptoms of Anxiety and Fear?

What happens when you become extremely anxious? Your body may react physiologically. You may become short of breath, your heart may beat rapidly, you may feel shaky, and you may think, "I've got to get out of here!" You may try to relax but be unable to do so. You may try to breathe deeply but find that the breath keeps catching in your throat. You may try to "shake the feeling" but find that you can't. This inability to calm down can be frightening, and may increase your anxiety even more. A vicious cycle can quickly develop. Before long, you may be completely out of control.

Which came first, the anxiety or the symptoms? That's not really important. What's more important is doing whatever is possible to reduce both. And it is possible to cope with fear—to regain control of your emotions and improve your day-to-day life.

## Is Fear Good or Bad?

Believe it or not, fear is usually good! Now, you're probably wondering how this is possible. Fear mobilizes you. It tells you to prepare to attack the source of your fear. You react in a way that leads to action. In this regard, fear is similar to stress. It serves a necessary and critical purpose. In a way, it protects you.

Anxiety is bad only when the source of your fear becomes overlooked, ignored, or denied, or when the feeling is so excessive that it paralyzes you. In such cases, the threat or danger is allowed to continue, and nothing—or, at least, not enough—is done to control it.

## What Determines the Intensity of Our Reactions?

Fear ranges in intensity from mild to severe. It is impossible to measure just how much fear there is in anyone's life. This varies from person to person and from time to time.

What determines how fearful you get? For one thing, how close is the feared object, person, or event? (Wouldn't you be more afraid if you were having major surgery within the next three days than if you were having it in thirty days?) How vulnerable are you? (Do you truly hate surgery, or are you just tired of having to spend time in the hospital?) Finally, how successful are you at defending yourself? (Can you calmly accept the fact that you're having surgery, or do you scream a lot?) These are just some of the factors that determine how you handle fear.

## How Can You Cope with Anxieties and Fears?

Obviously, the more fears you have, the more difficulty you'll experience in making a successful adjustment to your new situation. Recognizing your fears and learning how to deal with them will help you live more happily and comfortably. How? I was afraid you'd never ask! Let's look at some of the ways in which you can help yourself better cope with your fears.

### PINPOINT THE SOURCE OF YOUR FEARS

The first step in coping with your fears is to use the "pinpointing" technique discussed in chapter 18. Identify and list exactly what you're afraid of and exactly why you are afraid. Then think about what you can do to alleviate your fears. As you begin planning your strategies and gradually putting your plan into operation, you'll feel better and better.

## RELAX!

Because relaxation is the opposite of tension, the use of relaxation techniques can be very helpful in coping with anxieties and fears. As mentioned earlier, there are many types of relaxation techniques: progressive relaxation, meditation, autogenics, deep breathing, and more. Regardless of what is provoking your fear, learning to relax is an important part of improving emotional well-being. (Detailed information about relaxation techniques can be found in chapter 15.)

## DESENSITIZE YOURSELF

One great technique for conquering fear is called *systematic desensitization.* Using this technique, you gradually desensitize yourself—that is, make yourself less vulnerable—to the source of your fear.

Here's how it can work for you. Sit in a comfortable chair and relax. Then create a movie in your mind by imagining whatever it is that makes you afraid. If you get tense, stop imagining it and relax. When you've calmed down, try imagining it again. The more you try to imagine your fear, and alternate this "movie" with relaxation techniques, the less it will bother you. Try it! It will give you a great feeling of relaxation and control. There are many books that provide much more information on systematic desensitization. Check them out.

## LEARN TO COPE WITH ANXIOUS THOUGHTS

It was stated earlier that anxiety is a vague, uneasy feeling with an unknown source. So how can you cope with anxiety by following the steps listed above? Surely, if you can't pinpoint the source of your fear, you can't follow these specific steps. So what can you do? Well, a number of things may work. Try the relaxation techniques discussed in chapter 15. Work on changing your thinking to make it more positive and productive. Find somebody to whom you can express your fears—somebody who will listen to you, talk to you, and try to help you deal with your fears. Even if you can't pinpoint a specific fear, these techniques will greatly help you cope with general anxiety.

# When Are Antianxiety Medications Appropriate?

Many people are able to reduce anxiety through nonpharmacological methods such as those described on page 230. But if medication seems to be the answer for you—and especially if your anxiety is very intense—there are three subcategories that may be helpful.

The first subcategory of antianxiety drugs is the benzodiazepines. The drugs in this group include Xanax (alprazolam), Valium (diazepam), and Librium (chlordiazepoxide hydrochloride). The latter two, although used to control anxiety, are not considered as effective for panic attacks. Benzodiazepines have few side effects, but can be habit-forming.

The second subcategory of drugs primarily used in the treatment of anxiety is the tricyclic antidepressants. These medications were actually among the earliest ones found effective in dealing with anxiety but are now used less often, since more effective medications have been found. The drugs in this category include Tofranil (imipramine hydrochloride) and Norpramin (desipramine hydrochloride).

The third subcategory of antianxiety drugs is the MAO (monoamine oxidase) inhibitors. Some consider this group to be the most effective for in the treatment of anxiety. However, of the three groups, this one probably requires the greatest care in following dosage schedules and other precautions in order to minimize side effects. For example, if you're taking an MAO inhibitor, it is important to avoid taking antihistamines or decongestants, as the drugs might be incompatible and cause further problems. Also, foods with high concentrations of tyramine or dopamine—aged cheeses, beer, and wine, for instance—should be avoided, as they may lead to hypertension (high blood pressure). Examples of drugs in this subcategory are Nardil (phenelzine sulfate) and Parnate (tranylcypromine sulfate).

Because medication causes chemical changes within the body, side effects may occur whenever a drug is taken. And unfortunately, the more powerful the drug, the more potent its side effects may be. If the side effects you experience are slight, you will probably want to ignore them—

especially if the medication you're taking is having the desired effect. However, if side effects are very uncomfortable, talk to your doctor. Together you can weigh the disadvantages against the advantages. In fact, any side effects should be reported to your doctor so that he or she can determine if the drug therapy should be continued, changed, or ended.

When using antianxiety medications, keep in mind that even when they are effective, they are really only blocking the anxiety. It is still important to deal with the triggers of the fears and anxieties, and to implement any changes necessary to resolve the problems that led to the anxiety in the first place.

## Let's Talk About Specifics

When you were first diagnosed, many fearful questions probably came to mind. "What will the future be like? What will become of me?" These are all typical questions of people who are diagnosed with any chronic medical problem—not just diabetes.

As time has gone by, in all probability some of these questions have been answered and you have started to adjust to living with diabetes. But once your initial fears are reduced, new fears usually focus on more specific questions. In other words, you now focus on the fear that you won't master self-care, or the fear of long-term complications, or the fear of other possible events and experiences. All of these fears are normal and understandable, and should be expected. But however normal they may be, they can become extremely harmful if you fail to cope with them effectively.

In the previous pages, we looked at some general coping strategies. But you're probably more interested in seeing how these and other strategies can help you better deal with the specific fears that you're struggling with right now. Let's discuss some of these fears and see what methods of coping may help.

## FEAR OF NEEDLES

Fear of needles is very common, even for people who don't have diabetes. Lots of people are afraid of getting shots. Some put off going to doctor's appointments, because their dislike of needles is so intense. But if you need insulin, avoiding the use of needles is just not an option. You will have to overcome this fear for your health's sake.

The good news is that most people who take insulin report that the anticipation of taking insulin shots is much worse than actually taking the shots. The needles manufactured today are extremely fine and virtually painless. Additionally, your health-care team will be there to guide you as you learn to give yourself injections. Your doctor or diabetes educator will teach you safe and efficient ways to give yourself insulin shots so the process will be smooth and quick.

Millions of people with diabetes have learned to make insulin injections a regular part of their routine. There's no doubt that a great number of these people were afraid of needles before they became accustomed to using them. With time and patience, you can conquer your fear also.

## FEAR OF COMPLICATIONS

Fear of developing complications is very common among people with diabetes—and it's an understandable concern. Lots of people with diabetes are afraid they'll have to restrict their activities because of physical problems such as neuropathy or retinopathy. Many fear that they'll be disabled because of diabetes-related complications. These are certainly scary thoughts.

So how can you overcome this fear? Tell yourself that having diabetes doesn't mean complications are inevitable; even if they do occur, the effects may not be severe. And you're not going to develop complications just because you *think* it might happen!

In this case, fear can actually be a good motivator. If you're afraid of developing complications, perhaps you'll be more inspired to take good care of yourself, to really buckle down and control your diabetes (if you aren't already doing so!). Take life—and your diabetes management—one day at a time. Accept your condition, and do everything you can to keep your body healthy.

## FEAR OF DEPENDENCE

If you are finding that diabetes has placed some restrictions on your activities, you may be afraid of becoming too independent on your friends and family. You may worry that you'll be too much of a burden on your loved ones if you ask for help. You may fear that you'll lose your ability to help yourself.

You can deal with this fear by concentrating on those things that you still can do. Graciously accept the help you may have to take from others, but don't view this as dependence. Instead, focus on the benefits you're receiving from increased interaction with family and friends! So don't let yourself give up—you'll be doing yourself a great disservice.

## FEAR OF PAIN

Nobody likes pain. And because pain may develop as the result of a diabetes-related complication, you may be fearful of it. Each little twinge of pain may make you afraid—afraid that a more serious problem is developing. And even when you're not in pain, you may fear its occurrence.

What can you do about this fear? Try to accept the fact that you'll experience some pain from time to time, but that medication can reduce its intensity as well as its duration. Realize that each pain "cycle" will eventually stop, or at least ease up. The pain won't last forever. (For more suggestions on coping with pain, refer back to chapter 15.)

## FEAR OF "WHAT NEXT?"

What will happen next? Unfortunately, you can't be sure. Will you be able to keep your blood sugar level controlled? Will you develop any side effects from your medication? Will you have to deal with short- or long-term complications?

Everyone wonders what the future will hold. But because of the unpleasantness of what you're experiencing, you may be afraid of the future, rather than merely curious. What can you do? Because you can't foresee what will happen, take life one day at a time. Tell yourself that you'll handle any problems as they occur. Just keep doing what you have to do in order to take care of yourself.

## FEAR OF THE REACTIONS OF OTHERS

Are you afraid that others will shy away from you because you have diabetes? Unfortunately, some people can be cold and unfeeling. For example, they may be put off by the fact that you can no longer keep up with them. But your true friends will accept you under any circumstances.

Naturally, you should aim to remain involved with family and friends. But be realistic. Remember that a change in a social relationship can occur for any reason, not just because of diabetes! And since you can't change the way some people feel, try not to be too concerned with their reactions. Instead, be more attentive to your own needs and feelings.

Of course, if you feel that an important relationship is in jeopardy, you should try to figure out why and what you can do to improve things. And if you feel that people are shying away from you, try to discuss this with them. Find out what they are afraid of. Maybe you'll be able to remedy the situation. Get counseling, if need be. But remember that you can only do so much. If your efforts don't work, at least you'll know that you did your best.

Finally, if you have been troubled by the reactions of others, you may find it helpful to get involved in a support group. You know that the people in these groups will not shy away from you or abandon you. Why? Because they're going through the same kinds of things that you are! And because of their own experiences, participants may even be able to give you some tips on dealing with family and friends. (For more information on dealing with others, see chapters 26 to 30.)

## FEAR OF OVERDOING OR UNDERDOING

You may not know how much you should be doing. You may be afraid of doing too much, but feel guilty about doing too little! How can you conquer this fear? Get advice from experts. You'll need professional guidance to come up with the best "mix" of rest and exercise. And you'll need to know which, if any, activities may be too strenuous for you.

Of course, even your doctor may not have specific answers for you. You may be told that the answers will become apparent only through trial and error. After all, experience is the best teacher.

So what should you do? Pace yourself. Change your level of activity gradually. Then tell yourself, as with so many other fears, that you're doing the best you can.

## FEAR OF EMPLOYMENT PROBLEMS

Like many people with diabetes, you may be concerned about the effect your condition will have on your job. You may want or need to work, but fear that you won't be able to. Your employer may be understanding at first, but you may worry about how long his or her tolerance will continue. And, of course, your need for money will be greater due to your medical problems! So if you can't work, the pressure can be tremendous. (Refer to chapter 16 for more employment tips.)

What can you do? Talk to others who have been in the same situation, and see how they handled it. Speak to experts who can advise you on financial matters. Evaluate your vocational skills, and make sure you're equipped to do a job that you can physically handle. Remember, you'll work it out. (Look to chapter 17 for more advice on handling financial problems.)

## FEAR OF TRAVELING

People with diabetes don't have to limit their travel, but traveling with diabetes does present special circumstances and challenges. To some people with diabetes, the preparation required to take a "relaxing" vacation can be overwhelming. And the thought of traveling far from familiar doctors and medical facilities can be downright frightening. What if you run out of insulin? What if you lose your supplies? Who will take care of you if you get sick? What if you have an insulin reaction?

Proper planning can ensure that you have a fun and *safe* trip—to almost every corner of the globe! For example, always take more than enough insulin or oral diabetes medication along, just in case your return home is delayed. Carry your medications, supplies, testing materials, and glucagon with you at all times—even on the plane or train—so you'll have them when you need them. Research your destination to find out how to get medical care. The International Association for Medical Assistance to Travelers can provide information on doctors who speak your primary language. (Refer back to chapter 14 for more guidelines that will help ensure an enjoyable trip.)

### FEAR OF NOT COPING

You may feel that you're barely handling your diabetes. You may believe that any new problem that comes along will be enough to push you over the edge. And fear of falling apart can easily lead to panic: an out-of-control kind of feeling that can actually make this happen.

So get hold of yourself. Pinpoint those particular things you're having difficulty with, and get help in dealing with them. Don't wait, and don't project a false sense of bravado. If you feel yourself nearing the edge, get someone to help you to steady yourself. Talk over your fears with someone. Once you have shared them, you may see things a little more clearly. You may be able to deal with problems with greater strength, knowing that you're not alone. And once you're back in control, your fear will disappear.

## A Fearless Summary

Although many different fears have been discussed in this chapter, we probably haven't covered all of the ones you have experienced. In addition, the coping suggestions offered certainly don't include all possible ways of dealing with fear.

Anticipate that you will be fearful of certain things from time to time. Some fears will return, but plan on riding through them rather than succumbing to them. Not only is it okay to be scared, it's normal. Also remember that the most important thing is to stay on top of these fears so that they don't overwhelm you or render you less able to cope.

You're working on recognizing your fears, right? For some of them, you're modifying your behavior. For others, you're modifying your thinking. Soon you will feel more in control. As this happens, you'll notice your fears begin to diminish. That doesn't mean that they'll all go away. But as you work on them, they'll at least lessen in intensity, and you'll feel better knowing that you can handle whatever comes along.

# CHAPTER TWENTY-TWO

# Anger

Mary was fed up. She was tired of watching what she ate. She was annoyed at having to check her blood sugar every day. She was sick of giving herself insulin shots. From her doctor to her husband, practically everyone who went near her received an earful! Was Mary angry? You bet your eardrums she was!

In general, people with any chronic medical problem may be angry. These feelings are often exacerbated if the illness requires extra self-care. Because anger results in the buildup of physical energy that needs to be released—in other words, stress—it's important to learn how to cope with this emotion.

Just what is anger? When you have a desire or goal in mind and something interferes with your efforts to reach it, this can be very frustrating. A feeling of tension and hostility may result, which is what we refer to as anger.

# Are There Different Types of Anger?

In learning to deal with anger, it can be helpful to discuss the three different ways in which anger can be experienced. This will enable you to more easily identify anger when it does occur.

The first type of anger is rage—the expression of violent, uncontrolled anger. If Mary was feeling upset about her diabetes and a friend told her that she wouldn't be so uncomfortable if she didn't get so "worked up" all the time, you can imagine how angry Mary might become. Mary's anger might even lead her to say or do things that would certainly not enhance the prospects of a long-lasting, friendly relationship with this person! This is probably the most intense anger you can experience. It is an outward expression that results in a visible explosion. Often, rage can be a destructive release of the intense physical energy that has built up over time.

The second type of anger is resentment. This feeling of anger is usually kept inside. What if Mary listened to her friend's well-meaning comments, smiled, and said nothing, but was seething inside? This is resentment—a growing, smoldering feeling of anger directed toward a person or object but often kept bottled up. Resentment tends to sit uncomfortably within you and can do even more physiological and psychological damage than rage.

The third type of anger is indignation, a more appropriate, positive type of anger. Unlike rage, it is released in a controlled way. If Mary had responded to her friend's comments by stating that she appreciated the concern but would prefer no advice at this point, this would have been an expression of indignation.

Obviously, these three types of anger can occur in combination and in many different ways. Understanding the different ways of experiencing anger can help you identify and cope with it when it does occur.

## What Causes Anger?

There are, of course, lots of things that can make you angry. For some people with diabetes, the extra self-care that diabetes management requires can certainly be a source of anger. You may be angry because you can't eat what you want. You may become angry if you believe that your diabetes has imposed limitations on your life. You may get angry if you feel that your family is not understanding enough, or you may think that they are trying too hard to protect you. Or you can become frustrated if you can't seem to keep your blood sugar controlled no matter how hard you try—and this may cause you to feel angry.

Thoughtless comments from others can cause anger, as well. If you sense that someone is taking advantage of you, or if you feel forced to do something that you don't want to, anger may result. If you do not have the ability or confidence to say "no" when friends ask for a favor, this, too, can create feelings of anger—especially if you are feeling too fatigued to complete even your own tasks.

Becoming more aware of why you are angry is an important step in learning to deal with feelings of frustration or hostility. You must, of course, become aware of anger before you can deal with it. Unfortunately, resolving your anger won't make your diabetes go away. Nor should you say that you'll stop being angry only if your diabetes is cured. Neither attitude will help you.

One of the common questions that people with diabetes ask is "Why me?" This question suggests that what has happened shouldn't have happened—that it's unfair, or that someone or something is to blame. It's important to realize that in this case, anger is not helpful—that asking "Why me?" will not benefit you in any way. It's far better to ask yourself what you can do about it now that it has happened.

In learning to cope with your anger, you must realize that anger exists uniquely in the mind of each angry individual. Anger is a direct result of your thoughts, not of events. An event in and of itself does not make you angry. Rather, your anger is caused by your interpretation of the event—the way you think or feel about it.

## How Does Anger Affect Your Body?

When you are angry, a number of physiological responses occur. Your breathing becomes more rapid, your blood pressure increases (you may feel like your blood is "boiling"), and your heart may begin to pound. Your face may feel hot and your muscles may tense. You may also feel stronger when you're angry. The more intense the anger, the greater is this feeling of power. In fact, you may be able to remember a time when you were so angry that you almost felt you had superhuman strength.

Anger is a form of energy. The more physical energy that builds up in the body due to anger, the more necessary it becomes to release it. The energy cannot be destroyed. So if it is not released in some constructive manner, it will eventually come out in another, less desirable way.

Imagine the energy from anger as a stick of dynamite about to explode. If you get rid of it, it may cause some damage when it explodes, but it won't hurt you as much as it would if you swallowed it to keep others from getting hurt. Obviously, the ideal solution is neither to throw nor swallow the dynamite, but to defuse it. (More about defusing later on in the chapter.)

Extreme anger usually passes quickly. If, however, the anger lasts for a long period of time, it can have physically damaging effects on the body. You've probably heard about some of the physical problems that can result from holding anger in, such as ulcers, hypertension, and headaches. Well, anger can also affect your blood sugar levels. Because negative feelings such as anger put stress on your body, your blood sugar may be more difficult to control. So it's vital that you learn to deal with your anger, not just for your emotional well-being but for your physical health, as well.

## How Does Anger Affect Your Mind?

Anger is usually experienced as a very unpleasant feeling. However, it sometimes exists along with a more pleasant feeling of power or strength. Frequently, the unpleasantness of anger is related to its consequences—knowing what you do when you are angry, and not being happy about it.

Sometimes anger may become so extreme that you feel like exploding. You may feel that unless you are able to punch, kick, or hit something—to get rid of the anger in some way—you will lose control. Hopefully this angry energy can be released without causing damage to another person, property, or yourself. If, when you finally calm down, you find that you have done something destructive, you may become angry all over again. Or you may experience another negative emotion, such as guilt.

## Is Anger Good or Bad?

You may wonder how anger could possibly be good or constructive. "Avoid anger at all costs," many people say, "because nothing good can come of it." But this is true only if you don't deal with the anger properly. Anger can, indeed, be dangerous if it's kept inside or released in inappropriate ways.

Remember that stick of dynamite? What an explosive example! If anger is released in destructive ways, it can cause problems in relationships—to say the least! It can also aggravate existing medical problems. Does this mean that anger can make your condition worse? Well, what if you're so angry at somebody—perhaps your doctor or an overprotective spouse—that you don't follow your treatment program? "I'll show them," you say. This is obviously harmful, because you've turned your anger against yourself. And, in truth, you're only hurting yourself if you fail to keep your blood sugar levels under control.

How can anger be constructive? First, it can give you an indication that something is wrong—something that needs attention. Second, it can motivate you to deal more actively with life's problems. Anger can give you a feeling of power or strength, of confidence or assertiveness. This is not to say that you break a couple of dishes or have someone slap you in order to make you angry enough to solve your problems! What I am saying is that anger can be positive, and it can help you to solve problems.

## Some Different Reactions to Anger

Noreen, a forty-six-year-old teacher, was having a hard time with her husband. He was trying to show his concern by relieving her of all the responsibilities around the house. But she wanted to continue doing her household chores, and to be treated as normally as possible. She wanted to be the one to determine what she could and could not do. But Noreen's husband couldn't see this, and Noreen was running out of patience. Let's look at some ways in which this situation might be handled.

### THE "JUST IGNORE IT" APPROACH

If you feel overwhelmed by the intensity of your anger, and fear that you may completely lose control, you may try to do whatever you can to avoid the experience. This might include pushing any angry thoughts out of your mind, no matter how important the issue.

So rather than making a fuss over household responsibilities, Noreen could try to get involved in other activities and not show her resentment. Or she could try to appease her husband and agree with everything that he says. This would be at least temporarily effective in helping Noreen cope. In the long run, however, you can see that this would not be the best way for Noreen to deal with anger.

### THE "TAKE POWER" APPROACH

Maybe you enjoy the flow of energy and strength that comes from being angry. You may find that when you're angry, you are best able to assert yourself and get things done.

Noreen knows that if she is smothered once too often, she will explode. She might love the feeling of power that this anger gives her. She might almost look forward to the chance to say, "Honey, if you treat me that way once more, I'll take this vacuum cleaner and . . . !" If you enjoy this feeling, it's possible that you may even provoke situations to make yourself angry. Perhaps you've heard of professional football players or boxers who psyche themselves up before a confrontation with an opponent. For them, getting angry is the best preparation for a successful performance.

### THE "TAKE ACTION" APPROACH

It's possible to see anger as a necessary, though unpleasant, part of life. You know that there will be times when you'll be angry, whether you like it or not. But you can choose to deal with both your anger and the situation that's causing it as effectively as possible.

For example, Noreen knows that she's not happy being angry, and might decide to speak to her husband so that he could better understand her emotional needs. In this case, even if Noreen failed to persuade her husband to let her assume her normal household responsibilities, she would at least have the satisfaction of knowing that she did something about her feelings.

Your own reaction to anger is unique. It may also change from time to time. There may be times when you accept anger and almost value it as a motivator. At other times you may attempt to push it away. Noreen might enjoy expressing her anger. But if she didn't want to hurt her husband or upset the rest of the family, she might choose to have a calm discussion rather than shattering everyone's eardrums with an explosive confrontation.

Of course, the way in which you deal with your emotions now is probably similar to the way in which you've dealt with adversity in the past. If you have always dealt with problems in a generally positive, constructive manner, you will probably deal with new problems in the same way. On the other hand, if you have had difficulty dealing with stress in the past, you may also have problems dealing with it now. But remember that you *can* learn how to effectively cope with anger. Let's learn more about this.

## How Can You Cope with Anger?

You've now begun to realize that anger can be constructive. Hopefully, the information you've read so far has been encouraging. But what, specifically, can you do to cope with your own anger?

Because anger is such a complex emotion, and because so many things can lead to this feeling, there are no simple answers. (Sorry about that!) Does this mean that there is nothing that anybody can do about anger? No. Many things can be done to reduce your feelings of anger and to help you handle them more efficiently, comfortably, and safely.

First, of course, you must be able to admit that you're angry, and you must figure out why you're angry. Once you've pinpointed the source of your anger, you may be able to defuse it or, if that's not possible, to find an acceptable outlet for it. Let's take a look at each of these ways of coping with anger.

## RECOGNIZE YOUR ANGER

There are two steps involved in recognizing anger: admitting its existence and identifying its source. Let's discuss these in greater detail.

### *Step One: Admit That You're Angry*

The first step in dealing with anger is to recognize that you're angry. As simple as this may sound, many people cannot admit to being angry. They may try to deny it, or to rationalize their feelings or behaviors using other explanations.

Do you feel that being angry is a sign of weakness? If so, you may not admit that you're angry—perhaps not even to yourself. You may feel that there is no appropriate reason to be angry and that anger is a childish reaction. But, as with anything else, in order to change something, you have to first recognize that it exists.

How can you tell that you're angry? If you feel very tense (jumping at the sound of the telephone), or if you find yourself reacting with impulsiveness (slamming down the phone when you get a wrong number and storming out of the house) or hostility (cursing at your neighbor for leaving a speck of garbage on your lawn), chances are that you're angry. Don't be afraid to recognize it, as this is the first step in dealing with it.

### *Step Two: Identify the Source of Your Anger*

The second step in dealing with anger is trying to identify its source. Where did the anger come from? What is contributing to it? What events have led to these feelings of anger?

For one thing, as mentioned earlier in the chapter, you may be angry because you have diabetes. You may be angry with yourself for neglecting your condition. You may feel anger toward your physician, whether justified or not. You may be angry because you have to take insulin, or because you must monitor your blood glucose levels every day. In some cases, the events leading to an angry reaction may be quite obvious. In other cases, however, it may be hard to pinpoint the cause. At such times, be sure to probe deeply enough to find the source of the problem.

Once you've determined why you're angry, you want to decide whether the anger you're feeling is realistic. If necessary, write down what you think is making you angry. Be honest when writing down your thoughts, regardless of how violent or profane they may be! Rich, colorful language can be helpful in getting your feelings out, and will ultimately allow you to control your anger. Try to look at these thoughts objectively, the way someone else might look at them. If you recognize that your reasons are not rational, these alone may help you deal with your feelings. If, on the other hand, you can objectively say that your feelings of anger are rational, your next step will be to decide how you can best handle them.

Now, depending on the situation, you can either defuse your anger or find an appropriate outlet for it. Read on to see how each of these techniques can work for you!

## DEFUSE YOUR ANGER

In the past, it was falsely believed that there were only two possible ways of dealing with anger: to keep it inside or to let it out. But what about a third possibility? Remember when we talked about defusing that stick of dynamite? Your anger is a result of the way you think! In your mind, you're interpreting events in a way that makes you angry. So if you can change the way you interpret things and reorganize your thinking patterns, you can actually stop creating the anger that you feel. Is this really possible? Well, if something happened that made you angry, would everybody in the world be angry because of it? No. You'd be angry because of the way you'd be thinking about, or interpreting, the event. Others might not be angry because their interpretation of the event would be different. Let's look at some of the ways in which you can defuse your anger *before* it becomes a problem.

### *Watch Mental Movies*

When you become angry, you frequently have all kinds of pictures in your head—images of what's making you angry and of how you'd like to deal with your feelings. These "mental movies" can be helpful means of defusing your anger.

For example, imagine that you are very, very tired. Your friend calls to tell you that her car has broken down. Could you please pick her up? When you tell her that you are too exhausted to go out, she says something about how she can never depend on you for anything. This is a friend? You become irate. At that moment, ask your friend to hold on. Then close your eyes, and imagine all the abusive things that you would like to say to her. Then imagine the shocked expression on her face. By using mental imagery, you'll probably be able to complete the phone call without destroying a friendship. You may even smile or laugh as you think about the scenes playing through your mind.

Susan was quite fed up with her husband, Tom. Whenever she asked for his help around the house, he was grouchy and uncooperative. Just before Susan was about to lose it, she remembered the mental movie technique. Susan imagined herself strangling and clobbering Tom every time he talked back to her. This helped to rid Susan of the intense, angry feelings that were making her crazy, and allowed her to deal with Tom more constructively.

### *Picture a Big Red Stop Sign*

Another technique that can help you to control anger is "thought stopping." Remember: It is the thoughts in your mind that are making you angry—the thoughts you have when you interpret an event. So when you find that angry thoughts have come into your head, picture a big red stop sign. Seeing that picture in your mind will serve as a momentary distraction. Then concentrate on something you enjoy. This can be a peaceful, relaxing scene, an activity that you enjoy, or a favorite movie or television program. Whatever you choose, you will divert your thinking and give your anger a chance to dissipate. You could also participate in a pleasant activity—such as reading a book or taking a walk, for instance. Any of these activities should help defuse your anger.

### *Change Your Requirements*

At times, you may have specific requirements—particular ways in which you want certain things to occur. When these are not met, you may feel angry. Modifying your requirements can help you cope with your anger.

Let's say that you're not feeling well and you decide to call your doctor. The answering service tells you that she is not in the office and that you should get a return call within half an hour. After an hour, the doctor has not yet returned your call, and you are fuming. Why? Because your requirements were not met.

What can you do? Revise your requirement. Tell yourself that you would have liked a call within thirty minutes, but that your doctor may be tied up on another case, in transit, or simply unable to get to a phone. You'll be satisfied if you get a call at her earliest convenience. By modifying your requirement, you'll feel less angry.

Another way to benefit from this technique is to write down your requirements. Then try to revise them with new, more flexible desires. This may help you see your requirements in a more objective light.

### *Put Yourself in the Other Person's Shoes*

One of the best ways of dealing with anger toward somebody is to try to understand exactly what that person is feeling—what the person wants, or why the person is saying what he or she is saying. This will make you more aware of the reason for his or her behavior, and will also help you deal with it more constructively. Perhaps just as important, this technique can help you understand how that other person will feel if he or she is the target of an abusive release of anger.

## LET YOUR ANGER OUT

We have now discussed a number of ways in which you can control your thinking and improve your ability to interpret events in ways that will prevent anger from growing. But these techniques might not always be successful. What if there are times when you remain angry? What can be done to deal with anger constructively when it can't be defused? Fortunately, there are two possibilities.

### *Talk, Don't Bite*

Obviously, it is much more desirable to have a constructive discussion over an issue than an angry exchange of heated words that accomplishes nothing. In most cases, anger arises when you have a conflict or problem with another person. For this reason, it can be very helpful to learn how to get your point across constructively so that you can negotiate a solution. Remember that a heated argument—fighting fire with fire—is not the answer. Instead, you want to fight the fire by dousing it. In other words, you want to reduce the heat of the argument.

How can this be done? Try complimenting the person, or looking for positive things in what the person is saying to you. This will work in two ways. First, it will probably surprise the person. How will this help? Well, part of what fuels the fire of anger is your anticipation of the other person's anger. So by catching that person off guard, and thereby preventing him or her from reacting with anger, you will reduce this fuel. Second, by focusing on words or thoughts that are more constructive, you will calm yourself, rather than letting your anger grow. And once you're calm, you'll be able to quietly state your feelings.

### *Write Out Your Anger*

Write an angry letter. There are times when something or someone makes you so angry that you feel as if you're going to explode. You recognize the need to release these feelings because they're damaging to you, but either you don't trust yourself to speak to the person, or you don't have the confidence to speak up. This would be a great time to write an angry letter. Writing such a letter can be a constructive way of diffusing this intense anger, without damaging any relationships in the process. To whom should you write? You could write to your doctor, your partner, your neighbor, the medical profession, the "powers above"—virtually anyone, real or not, with whom you feel angry. But remember that for this technique to work best, you can't let anyone see your letter! After you finish pouring your heart onto paper, destroy it. You'll be destroying some of your anger at the same time.

### *Find a Physical Release for Your Anger*

In general, one of the best outlets for releasing your anger is physical activity. Some people find that they can release the physical energy from anger by *watching* things! For example, by watching a sporting event, you may not be releasing energy through participation in the sport, but you may be able to release anger by "getting into" the activities you're viewing. Or you might want to try watching an emotionally draining movie. You may become so totally absorbed that your built-up energy is released through worry, fear, or excitement. A book that allows you to identify with the characters can be beneficial as well—especially if the characters themselves release anger.

Believe it or not, another common and very effective outlet for anger is crying. You've probably heard about the therapeutic effects of a good cry. However, this technique is not for everyone. For instance, you may think that it's "immature" to cry—although you might be amazed by the number of people who unashamedly let their tears flow. But if your anger has built up to the point of uncontrollable crying, this will be a great way to let it out. (Of course, you may scare the daylights out of your family. But just tell them you read about it here!)

Some people like to count to ten when angry. This may distract you from what is making you angry, giving you a chance to calm down and think about it more constructively. Try counting out loud, and expressing your feelings through facial expressions and tone of voice. Count to a thousand, if necessary!

## An Anger-Free Summary

As you learn to cope with your anger, it's important to remember that events alone do not make you angry. It is your thinking—your interpretation of these events—that leads to anger. And since it is your thinking that makes you angry, you are responsible for feeling this way. Therefore, you are just as responsible for changing your thinking to help yourself cope with anger—or at least to reduce it to a more manageable level.

The best way to handle anger is probably to be in control so that it doesn't build up in the first place—to restructure your thinking so that your emotions don't get out of hand. But if anger does build, remember that when it is channeled and used constructively, it can be beneficial. And when this isn't possible, you can defuse or release your anger in a harmless way.

# CHAPTER TWENTY-THREE

# Guilt

Have you ever felt guilty? Many individuals with diabetes say that they have. Certainly, this is a very unpleasant feeling. You may feel guilty because treatment for diabetes costs money. You may feel guilty if you don't stick to your diet, or if you don't exercise as often as you should. Or you may experience guilt because of feelings you have toward other people—resentment, perhaps, or jealousy—because they don't have diabetes.

It may not be easy to cope with guilt, but you don't have to let yourself become a victim of these feelings. Let's first take a look at what leads to guilty feelings, and then explore some ways in which you can reduce your feelings of guilt. After all, you want to do everything possible to make yourself feel better, and it's hard to feel good when you're feeling guilty!

## What Are the Two Components of Guilt?

Feelings of guilt usually have two components. The first of these is the sense of *wrongdoing*—the feeling that you have either done something wrong or haven't done something that you should have done. The second component is the feeling of *badness* that results from the self-blame. It's this second component that's the true culprit! When you feel bad about doing something wrong, this is normal and understandable. But when you start telling yourself that you are a bad person, guilt follows.

## What Causes Guilt?

There are lots of things you might feel guilty about, even though there's probably no validity to any of them. For example, maybe you're concerned about something you did to contribute to the development of your diabetes. You may, for instance, feel guilty because you didn't take care of yourself properly, perhaps eating too many unhealthy foods and allowing yourself to become overweight. Perhaps you feel that if it weren't for certain actions—or lack of actions—on your part, you would not be in this situation. You may also feel guilty because you believe that you're complicating things for your family. Therefore, you blame yourself.

Perhaps others have told you that your feelings of guilt have no rational basis, that you're not at fault. Unfortunately, this may not eliminate guilt. Why? Because your feelings may have nothing to do with what others say or think. Remember: Your guilt comes from your own belief that you are a bad person.

Obviously, guilt can be a destructive emotion. It can drain you physically and emotionally, and can undermine your efforts to cope successfully with diabetes. Fortunately, there's plenty you can do to improve your outlook. In the remainder of this chapter, we'll look at the various techniques you can use to cope with guilt.

## How Can You Cope with Guilt?

Regardless of the cause of your guilt—and whether it is a new or longstanding problem for you—there are a number of strategies that can help you reduce or eliminate this unpleasant and harmful emotion. Let's take a look at some of the best ways of coping with guilt.

## FIND THE SOURCE OF YOUR GUILT

In order to successfully cope with guilt, you must first focus on what led to the guilty feelings in the first place. Sometimes, just by pinpointing the source of this emotion you can greatly reduce or even eliminate it.

First, ask yourself if you have actually done something wrong. If you feel you have, ask yourself if the behavior you're blaming yourself for was really that terrible. If you feel guilty because of your diabetes, ask yourself if that makes sense. Did you make it happen? Of course not. So identify the cause of your guilt and examine the wrongdoing you feel you committed. You will probably find either that you are not responsible for the wrong action, or that the action was really not terrible enough to justify your feeling so bad!

Sometimes people feel guilty about thoughts or desires, rather than specific actions or behaviors. Recognize the difference between feeling guilty over a thought and feeling guilty over an action. Then, once you've identified the thought that's making you feel like a bad person, change it. Learn to talk to yourself in a positive way. Look at thoughts objectively and constructively in order to reduce your guilt.

But what if you feel guilty and simply can't remember what you were thinking or doing that made you feel this way? How can you use all the great thought-changing ideas we're going to talk about if you can't identify the thoughts you want to change? Good question! In order to pinpoint these "target" thoughts or behaviors, you might want to keep a brief written log of feelings or activities that may be causing your guilt. Once you have written these down, you can begin to determine the root of the problem and then think about what changes might improve the situation.

## TALK IT OVER

It's very important to discuss how you feel about your condition with others who may be affected by it. Share your concerns, and try to figure out solutions to any problems that exist.

Janet, a fifty-two-year-old woman married for over twenty years, enjoyed the weekly dinner club she and her husband attended with other couples in their neighborhood. Now, because of necessary changes in her diet due to diabetes, she didn't want to struggle with all the different restaurants, and chose not to go out as frequently. She was afraid that she would go and eat too much, and then feel guilty that she was not taking care of herself. Sometimes, she didn't want to go out even once during an entire month. Not only did she feel unhappy about her condition, but she also felt extremely guilty about holding her husband back. She felt that he couldn't have a good time because of her. It would have been helpful for Janet to discuss alternatives with her husband. If she had arrived at a solution with her husband's cooperation, she could have effectively reduced her guilt feelings.

Fortunately, Janet had the good sense to sit down with her husband and discuss the situation. Janet felt better knowing that her limitations would not prevent her husband from enjoying social activities.

## TURN YOUR THOUGHTS AROUND

Is there anything you can do about the negative thoughts that lead to guilt—those thoughts that make you feel that you're a bad person? One helpful thing to do is to try to restructure your thinking to make it more positive and guilt-free.

For example, let's say that you feel guilty because you believe that you're not being a good parent. Ask yourself if you've ever done anything that a good parent might do. Just about every mom or dad can come up with something! This type of thinking will begin to eliminate your feelings of guilt. The idea is to turn your mind's negative thoughts into reasonable, positive ones. This way, the feelings of guilt will not take a stranglehold!

## REEVALUATE YOUR GOALS

Among the most common causes of guilt are thoughts containing the word "should"—"I *should* have been able to finish that job today" or "I *should* have taken my kids to the park today." These thoughts imply that you must be just about perfect and on top of everything. Naturally, you will become upset whenever you fall short of your "should." But should you blame yourself when "should" thoughts establish goals that are unrealistic—goals that you may not be able to fulfill? Of course you shouldn't!

Do you see a difference between the way you are doing something and the way you think you should be doing it? If so, you are probably feeling guilty! How can you work this out? Can you work harder or do more? If you can, and it's appropriate for you to do so, then you've solved your problem. If not, try examining your day-to-day goals for working and living. Ask yourself if these goals are practical, considering what you can and cannot do because of your diabetes.

So what steps can you take to stop feeling guilty about the things you *should* have done? For starters, reword your thoughts to eliminate the word "should." Use less demanding ones. Say, "It would be nice if I could finish that task today, but I can't," rather than, "I should finish that task today." If you have trouble changing the wording of your "should" thoughts, try asking yourself, "Why should I . . . ?" or "Who says I should . . . ?" or "Where is it written that I should . . . ?" This may help you decide whether you are setting up impossible requirements for yourself. It can also help you reduce your feelings of guilt.

Let's say, for example, that you are thinking of having a party because all your friends have invited you to get-togethers. Ask yourself why you should. Is it because the "Party Rulebook" tells you that otherwise your friendship license will be revoked? Is it because if you don't have a party, your friends—some friends!—won't invite you to their homes anymore? As you think of some realistic answers to these questions, you'll come to realize that you don't have to have a party. Although it would be nice, it would be more sensible to wait until you're feeling better.

Another way to eliminate guilt feelings over "should" thoughts is to take more pride in what you can do, rather than focusing on things you feel you should do but that you might not be up to. Although most people hate hearing that "things could be worse," this is quite true. There are people who can't do anything at all. If you concentrate on the things you can do, and dwell less on what you can't, your feelings of guilt will diminish and you'll feel a lot better. Changing the emphasis in your thinking will also help you lessen the perceived gap between what is and what you feel "should" be—which is what led to your guilty feelings in the first place.

### ESCAPE FROM ESCAPE BEHAVIOR

Sometimes, people who feel guilt—and have failed to cope with this destructive emotion—act in negative ways to hide from their feelings. There may be a tendency to indulge in "escape" behaviors, such as drinking or excessive sleeping. Instead of dealing with them head-on, they push them away.

Frank, a forty-seven-year-old contractor, felt guilty because he was not able to work as efficiently at his job as in years past. As a result, he earned less money and was not able to provide all of the luxuries he and his family would have otherwise enjoyed. In an attempt to "escape" and forget his misery, Frank started drinking. This behavior surely did not help the situation—in fact, drinking alcohol was downright dangerous to his health. And, as he drank more, his relationships with his wife and children became strained. The effects of his escape behavior only increased Frank's feelings of guilt, starting a vicious cycle.

As you may have already guessed, the first step toward improvement is to look past the escape behavior and identify what is causing the guilt. Then consider what can be done to rectify the problem. At the same time, try to eliminate the escape behavior, recognizing that this activity is not improving your situation in any way. If you have difficulty eliminating this behavior by yourself—or, for that matter, identifying the root of the problem—by all means consider working with a supportive professional. You're worth it!

It is possible, of course, that there is no clear-cut way to eliminate the situation or feelings that have led to your guilt. But don't give up. Instead, look for partial solutions. These may not be as desirable as complete solutions, but they can still help reduce your guilt and make you feel better about yourself.

## A Guiltless Summary

Guilt is a very destructive emotion—one that can interfere with your success in coping with diabetes, by lowering your self-image and exhausting your emotional resources. By becoming aware of how guilt develops, by pinpointing the source of your guilt, and by changing your thinking to be more positive and realistic, you should be able to decrease or eliminate this feeling, and instead use your energy to successfully cope with your condition.

# CHAPTER TWENTY-FOUR

# Stress

Stress! Every time you turn around, you either read or hear about stress. What exactly is it? Stress is a response that occurs in your body. It is a form of energy—a normal reaction to the demands of everyday life. It helps mobilize your strength to deal with different events and circumstances.

Many things occur each day that require you to adapt. These are known as *stressors*. The changes that take place in your body when something (the stressor) provokes you are known as the *stress responses.*

We all know that stress can play a role in causing or exacerbating virtually any medical problem. And diabetes is no exception. In fact, any experience with diabetes both causes and can be affected by stress.

## What Are the Symptoms of Stress?

Your body will tell you when the stress you're experiencing is excessive. What might you feel? Physically, excessive stress can manifest itself as sweaty palms, heart palpitations, tightness of the throat, fatigue, nausea, diarrhea, or headaches—among other things. Emotionally, depression, anxiety, anger, frustration, or simply a vague uneasiness are just a few possible symptoms. As long as you tune into your body and mind, you'll know when you can benefit from stress-reduction techniques.

## How Does Stress Affect You?

The effects of stress—much like the effects of depression, discussed in chapter 20—are not isolated problems. Instead, they are part of a complex response that can affect both your body and your emotions. Let's examine this in more detail.

### HOW STRESS AFFECTS YOUR BODY

Stress is a natural survival response. It occurs within the body whenever you feel threatened by thoughts or external stressors.

Stress can manifest itself in many ways. When you are in a stressful situation, your circulatory system speeds up and blood is pushed rapidly toward different parts of the body—particularly those organs and systems necessary to protect you—raising your blood pressure. Because the blood supply has been diverted, the supply to the digestive system is usually reduced as well, making the process of digestion slower and less effective. Stress also constricts the blood vessels, increases heart rate, and produces other physiological manifestations—all instantaneously!

What else can occur? You may tremble or perspire. Your face may flush. You may feel a surge of adrenaline flowing through your body. Your mouth may become dry and you may feel nauseated. Your breathing may become more rapid and shallow. Your heart may begin to pound. Your muscles may become tight, leading to headaches or cramps. Sounds wonderful, doesn't it?

So when you experience stress, your body prepares itself physiologically to counter any threat to its survival. Why? Well, perhaps you've heard of the *fight or flight* response. You see, when an animal feels threatened, it prepares to either fight or run away. You will never see an animal standing there, scratching its head and thinking about how it might best handle the situation! Even though we have the ability to think and reason, we also experience the fight or flight response, which causes the secretion of many different hormones and tenses the muscles in preparation for battle. If the response does involve physical action—fight or flight—the hormones are utilized as they are supposed to be, and the muscles are exercised, with energy being appropriately released. However, if there is no physical exertion—if you think instead of taking action—the energy that was mobilized may not be released in the way expected. This may explain why, after a period of stress during which no action was taken, you feel exhausted just the same.

When does stress lead to physical problems? When you can't respond to stress in a way that eliminates it, the stress continues unabated—and so do its symptoms. An inability to do anything to relieve the stress may cause even more stress, creating a vicious cycle. And this can take its toll on your body. In fact, many researchers believe that prolonged stress puts such a strain on your body that your immune system may ultimately break down, making your body more vulnerable to a number of diseases.

## HOW STRESS AFFECTS YOUR DIABETES

Stress is particularly dangerous for people with diabetes. The hormones that the body releases as part of the fight or flight response are meant to prepare the body for quick action. These hormones break down stored glycogen into blood glucose, which the body should be able to use for energy. But, as you know by now, people with diabetes can't effectively use this extra glucose for energy, so the result is a rapid rise in blood sugar.

During times of stress, your self-care skills slip a little bit. When you're under pressure—for example, if you have to meet a tight deadline—you may not take time to eat. Even if you do eat, chances are you won't spend too much time choosing healthy foods that fit into your diet plan. Or maybe you'll decide to forego exercise, because there are just too many other important things on your "to do" list. Some people like to have a few drinks to relax when they're feeling stressed. As we discussed in earlier chapters, any of these behaviors can seriously affect your blood sugar levels.

As if life weren't stressful enough, just the experience of having diabetes can be pretty stressful, too. You may feel under a great deal of pressure to maintain "perfect" control of your diabetes. You may feel stressed because sexual side effects of diabetes are interfering with intimacy. If you've detected some symptoms of a possible diabetes-related complication, you'll probably feel pretty wound up until you know all the facts.

### HOW STRESS AFFECTS YOUR MIND

Your emotional response to stress may not be as visible as your physical response. You may start worrying, and fear the next "event." Your attention span may be reduced, and you may be less able to concentrate on the task at hand. You may have trouble learning something new. You may be afraid to do things. You may withdraw or feel nervous. You may lose confidence in yourself.

As you become nervous and upset, you may become more aware of any unpleasant physical responses you're experiencing, and this may make you feel even more stressed. For example, if you have responded to stress with shallow, rapid breathing or heart palpitations, your awareness of these physical responses may lead to feelings of panic. Most people respond to stress both physically and emotionally, although it is possible to respond in only one way. Don't you have your own "typical" reaction? Maybe you become too jittery and unfocused to concentrate on your job. Perhaps you feel physically ill, with extreme intestinal discomfort or a throbbing headache. Regardless of what you feel, it's important to learn strategies that will enable you to deal effectively with stress.

## Three Reactions to Stress

We've just discussed how your body and mind respond to stress. But we also want to look at a third type of response—the way you choose to deal with stress.

When a stressful stimulus occurs, you will most likely react in one of three ways. You might not respond at all, and either "go with the flow" or become unable to function. You might respond immediately and impulsively without giving thought to whether a better response might be possible. Or you might respond to stressors in a well-planned, organized, and effective manner. If so, you may not even need this chapter! But if not, read on.

## Is Stress Good or Bad?

By now, you've probably figured out that stress can be either good or bad. It is good when it gives you extra energy to do the things that need to be done during stressful times. In fact, a certain amount of stress is normal and necessary. Stress helps you to "get your act together," and prepares you to handle your life in the best possible way. But when left unchecked, stress can be highly destructive, draining all of your energy and possibly worsening any existing physical or emotional problems. So while stress can be helpful, this chapter concerns itself with harmful stress—the kind that can hurt you if it goes uncontrolled.

## What Causes Stress?

A number of things can act as stressors. Work-related problems, marital disputes, family deaths, even some positive events—all can cause stress. But in this book, we're most concerned with the effects of diabetes on your life, and this can cause stress in a number of different ways. Problems with your treatment program or adjustments to dietary changes can cause stress. Fears of short- or long-term complications are also common stressors for people with diabetes. And worries about being able to fulfill responsibilities may provoke a stress response, as well.

Everyone has a unique way of responding to the world. Your pattern of response depends on a number of things. Your upbringing, your self-esteem, your beliefs about yourself and the world, the way in which you guide yourself in your thoughts and actions—all of these things help determine your stress response. The degree to which you feel in control of your life also plays an important role in this response. And the way you feel, physically and emotionally—as well as the way you get along with people—is also a factor.

To sum it up, everyone's method of dealing with stress is unique and individual, and depends on a complex combination of thoughts and behaviors. To keep things simple, though, we can view the stress response as dependent on the "chemistry" between two factors. The first factor is the stressor, or the outside pressure. In other words, what is going on around you that is creating a problem. The second factor is your interpretation of the event. It is the interaction of the stressor and your internal interpretation that determines your response to stress. (Sound familiar? Yes, it's the same "formula" that can be applied to anger, depression, and any other emotion.) So the "equation" for the stress response is as follows:

**Stressor + Interpretation = Stress Response**

This equation has important implications for coping with stress. Why? It shows you that stress is not solely the result of your environment, your illness, or any other factor around you. The way you interpret this stressor is of equal importance. Of course, some stressors would produce stress in anybody. What would happen, for example, if somebody pointed a knife at your throat? Calm acceptance, or a stress response? Get the point? In many situations, though, you do have the ability to control your reaction to the stressor.

As you learn to cope with stress, it's important to remember that your mind responds to any thoughts of stress as though they are real and happening right now. Any thoughts or images in your mind that produce a stress response are perceived as existing in the present, as the brain and nervous system do not recognize the difference between past, present, and future. So it's easy to see that you contribute to your body's stress response with your own thoughts and images. This makes it even more important to feed your mind with the best, most beneficial, and most constructive information available.

# How Can You Cope with Stress?

Because stress can affect the body and mind in so many ways, stress management is a very important part of any program for coping with diabetes. It's clear that stress can affect certain aspects of diabetes, including blood sugar levels. The good news is that, regardless of how successfully you have dealt with stress in the past, you can learn effective strategies that will help you deal with it now. These strategies will make you feel more in control, lessening the feelings of panic and increasing your emotional well-being.

But before we look at how you should cope with stress, let's look at what you *shouldn't* do. Smoking, alcohol abuse, the use of inappropriate drugs, and overeating are all common but poor coping strategies. True, these activities will distract you and perhaps delay the effects of the stress, but they can also hurt you and prevent you from coping with stress in a constructive way.

So what should you do? Try to learn new, more appropriate ways of dealing with stress. Relaxation techniques and regular exercise can be helpful parts of stress-management programs. And by thinking more appropriate and positive thoughts, you can go a long way toward reducing stress as well. But be realistic and remember that while stress can be managed and controlled, it cannot be eliminated. Your focus, then, should be on using the following management techniques to help yourself deal better with both the physical and the emotional effects of the stress response.

## USE RELAXATION TECHNIQUES

Because relaxation is incompatible with stress, the best way to start controlling stress is to use relaxation techniques. In fact, relaxation techniques alone—used without any other coping strategies—may allow you to successfully cope with both the physical and the emotional effects of stress.

Relaxation benefits you in many ways. First, it can give your body a chance to rest and recuperate. And a stronger body can help you deal better with the ravages of stress—and life! Relaxation will help you sleep better. Relaxation is also pleasurable, and will increase your feeling of emotional well-being. And it can give you a powerful sense of reestablishing control over your life, despite the presence of a chronic medical problem.

There are many different types of clinical relaxation techniques, including meditation, autogenics, and deep breathing. Hypnosis and biofeedback can also be used to induce relaxation, although they have other uses as well. (See chapter 15 for a full discussion of these and other relaxation techniques.)

One relaxation technique that is often successful in combating stress is imagery—a technique that can also be used to cope with pain and other problems. Imagery is the process of formulating mental pictures or scenes in order to harness your body's energy and improve your physical or emotional well-being. In this case, of course, you'll want to conjure up images that are relaxing and stress-free. Imagine not only the sights but also the smells, the tactile sensations (touch), and the sounds. The more vivid your image, the more helpful it will be. Feel comfortable with whatever degree of clarity your image takes on. The degree of relaxation you'll experience is up to you, and will benefit only you. You are in control.

## PINPOINT THE SOURCE OF YOUR STRESS

Now that you're more relaxed, you're ready to objectively identify your stressors. What, specifically, is causing you to feel stress? Maybe you're having a hard time with the symptoms of diabetes. Maybe you're tired of sticking to your treatment program. Or maybe you're just tired of thinking about diabetes. Of course, there are many more possibilities.

What if you're not sure what's causing your stress? Try keeping a log of your daily stressors. This will allow you to more easily recognize the people, places, and things that have the potential to create stress in your life. But what if you can't pinpoint which of your many activities are the real culprits? As you keep your log, you might want to use a numerical rating scale, such as the Subjective Units of Disturbance (SUD) scale. How does it work? Ratings on this scale range from 0 to 100, depending on the amount of stress you're experiencing. Use 100 to represent the most extreme and disturbing stress, and 0 to represent no stress—total and complete relaxation. Then rate your activities, experiences, and thoughts. The ones with the higher SUD numbers are the ones causing you the most stress. (For example, loud music blasting from your neighbor's radio might be rated a whopping 85!)

## IDENTIFY YOUR STRESS REACTIONS

Once you have begun identifying your stressors, you'll want to become completely aware of your responses to them. Are they more physiological or psychological? What parts of your body seem to be the most vulnerable? What kind of reactions does your body have? Does your attention span suffer? Do you get heart palpitations? Do you start losing confidence, or feel as if you're "slipping"? As you become more aware of these things, you will develop a complete picture of your own unique stress response. This picture will help you choose the coping strategies that will be most useful in dealing with your stressors.

## ELIMINATE STRESSORS WHEN POSSIBLE

What's the next step? Once you recognize which stressors are causing the most trouble, try to determine whether you can eliminate them. Removing the source of stress is an obvious and logical way to manage it. For instance, if the task of managing your household expenses is causing you stress, you might have your spouse take over this chore. Obviously, different types of stressors would have to be removed in other ways.

## CHANGE YOUR VIEW OF THE STRESSOR

What happens if you can't eliminate the source of your stress? You'll then have to work on your interpretation of the stressors. You might want to use some of the suggestions discussed in chapters 20 and 22. Or you might want to try systematic desensitization, discussed in chapter 21.

Another technique that might help you cope better with stressors is *stress inoculation.* How can you be inoculated against stress? Well, you're certainly familiar with the use of inoculations to protect children from diseases such as measles. By exposing a child to the virus or other agent that causes a disorder, inoculations gradually strengthen the child's immunity to the disorder. Similarly, stress inoculation uses mental rehearsal procedures to help you confront and gradually tolerate stressful situations. As we previously discussed, because your mind responds to thoughts and mental images as if they were real and happening right now, thinking about something can be just as stressful as experiencing it. So by learning to cope with a situation in your mind, you can learn how to cope with it before it even happens.

Start your stress inoculation process by using whatever relaxation techniques you have found most helpful. Once you have achieved a comfortable level of relaxation, start imagining one of the stressors you've previously identified. As you imagine the stressful scene, recognize any physiological sensations or psychological changes that you may be experiencing.

Margaret realized that much of her stress was being caused by the fear that, during an office visit, her doctor would tell her she had developed a long-term complication, such as neuropathy. Margaret's stress reaction—nausea and a tightening in her throat—would appear whenever she imagined this frightening scene. So she decided to use stress inoculation to gain control. Repeatedly she imagined herself in the very situation she feared. She visualized the doctor's office. She imagined herself sitting in the chair by the doctor's desk. She actually heard the words she was afraid of. As Margaret gradually increased her tolerance of this image, the symptoms of her stress lessened.

Like Margaret, whenever you use stress inoculation to visualize and mentally experience a scene, you'll increase your ability to handle that particular stressor, and your symptoms will decrease. In other words, your body and mind will be "inoculated," allowing you to tolerate that stressor. One added advantage of using this technique is that you will become more aware of exactly when these tension-producing situations begin to affect you. This will enable you to use your coping strategies sooner, before your body and mind begin suffering from the stress response.

If you have already read the explanation of systematic desensitization found in chapter 21, you may realize that stress inoculation and desensitization are very similar. But there is a difference. In desensitization, the technique of imagining a stressful situation is alternated with the use of relaxation techniques. In stress inoculation, relaxation techniques are employed only at the start of the session. Experimentation will show you which method is best for you.

## USE PHYSICAL STRESS RELIEVERS

Certain physical activities can be a great means of stress control. For example, some people relieve tension or stress by driving. Certainly, as long as you continue to observe safety rules—and as long as you enjoy this activity—driving can be very relaxing. But if driving isn't your idea of a calming pastime, there are a number of other activities that may be just the ticket.

### *Exercise*

Exercise is not only a wonderful means of releasing stress, but as you learned in chapter 9 it can be a very beneficial part of your diabetes treatment program. Regardless of how diabetes is affecting you, there is certain to be a type of exercise that will help you control your level of stress. Brisk walking, swimming, and dancing, for instance, all allow for the release of tension. Just be sure to get your doctor's approval before beginning any exercise program.

### *Keep Busy the Fun Way*

Hobbies and other leisure activities are often very effective ways to reduce stress. They can divert your attention from the stressful situation and direct it toward something more enjoyable. They may also help you to feel more productive—and a lack of productivity may be one of the stressors giving you problems in the first place! If you don't have a hobby, this is a great time to look into painting, model building, gardening—whatever suits your fancy. If you're already involved in a hobby, you now have the perfect reason to indulge yourself whenever you can.

### *Catch Up on Your Sleep*

Another technique for dealing with stress is sleep. Some people have difficulty sleeping when they're experiencing high levels of stress. But, when possible, catnaps or even prolonged periods of sleep may help you reduce stress to a more manageable level. After all, you need your rest anyway!

## A Stress-Free Summary

What are your goals? Are you trying to gain greater control over your emotions? Do you want to live life more fully? Whatever they are, if stress is keeping you from reaching them, then your stress response is negative. By learning how to control your stress—by eliminating the things that are stressing you, or by modifying your reaction—you'll be far more likely to meet these goals. Just as important, you'll have a head start in coping successfully with diabetes.

# CHAPTER TWENTY-FIVE

# Other Emotions

The emotions discussed in chapters 20 through 24 are not the only ones you may experience, of course. What other emotions might you want to learn to deal with better? This chapter will discuss three additional emotions that many people with diabetes have found to be problematic: boredom, envy, and loneliness.

## Boredom

Hopefully, by this time, you are not so bored that you have stopped reading! If I've still got your attention, let's talk a bit about boredom.

What an empty feeling boredom is! It's one of the worst feelings you can possibly experience. It has been said that more problems and tragedies are caused by boredom than by any other single emotion. I bet you never thought of diabetes as being boring. But it can be, primarily because of the restrictions your condition may impose on you. Some activities that provided enjoyment for you in the past may now be out of reach.

So what should you do? To begin with, don't let your condition cause you to give up on life. Distinguish between what you can do and what you can't. If you do have to curtail any activities because of diabetes, you'll do so. If you have to drop an activity, you'll drop it. But you don't have to eliminate all activities simply because you may not be able to complete them. How else can you fight the boredom blues? Read on!

## TRY NEW ACTIVITIES

If boredom is a problem for you, you'll certainly want to find ways to add some interest to your life. You may find that the activities you used to enjoy now seem artificial and uninteresting. You may no longer derive any pleasure from them. Don't feel that you must push yourself to enjoy these activities, as forcing yourself to be amused rarely works. Instead, try to find some new activities that will make your life more interesting. Remember that preferences change. Be open-minded, and try things that never appealed to you before. This time around, they may spark your interest.

## LEARN SOMETHING NEW

One of the most effective weapons against boredom is learning. The mind is like a sponge, always thirsty to soak up information and knowledge. Select a potentially interesting topic you don't know much about. Go out and learn something about it. You may want to begin by going to the library and reading some books on the topic. Perhaps you'd like to enroll in an adult education course. Boredom often disappears once you become involved in something new. As an added benefit, your new pursuit may put you in contact with some interesting new people. And increasing your circle of friends is always a good way to fight boredom.

## SET GOALS

Boredom often arises from plodding along with no purpose in life. So one of the best ways to fight it is to always give yourself something to look forward to—a goal. This doesn't mean that you'll never be bored. You may still have to give yourself an occasional kick in the butt to get yourself moving toward those goals. But the promise of some pleasurable activity will make it much easier to keep yourself going.

What kinds of goals might you set? They can be as simple as reading a chapter of a good book, writing a letter, making that phone call you've been thinking about, watching a television program you enjoy, or meeting somebody special for lunch. Try to schedule something to look forward to every day. This way, even if part of your day seems boring, you won't give the weeds of boredom a chance to take root!

## Envy

You've heard the cliché "The grass is always greener . . ." If you have diabetes, you are probably envious of those who don't. This is understandable. But envy is still a destructive emotion because it's a type of self-torture. When you feel envious, you're constantly putting yourself down and comparing your own qualities with the seemingly better qualities of somebody else. You feel inferior. And this can lead to other negative emotions, such as anger or depression.

Envy is often irrational. When you're envious, you want to be like somebody else. You want to have what somebody else has. Does this mean that the other person has a life that's happier than yours in every way? Stop and think for a moment. I'm sure you can come up with some areas in which your life is better!

### WHAT LEADS TO ENVY?

Basically, there are four conditions necessary for envy to occur. First, you must feel deprived in some way. You will feel like you can't have something that you want or need. I'm not talking simply about money, pleasure, or even health! Envy is an intense feeling that involves much more than this. It seems as if your feeling of need lies deep inside.

Second, to experience envy you must feel that somebody else has what you're missing. Perhaps the person has a bigger house, for instance. Or perhaps the person does not need to take insulin shots.

Third, you must feel powerless to do anything about this problem. You must feel totally unable to change the circumstances that have made you envious in the first place. This helplessness causes you to become more and more bitter. And this makes you even more envious!

Fourth, there must be a change in the relationship between you and the person whom you envy. You are no longer simply comparing yourself with that person; you now feel fiercely competitive. You may begin to feel that the only reason you don't have what you want is that somebody else has it.

There are two types of things that may cause you to feel envy. One type is tangible—jewelry, cars, homes, and so on. The other type is less tangible—friends, pleasure, or health, for instance. If you have diabetes, you may still have many tangible things. You may still have a car and a place to live. You may still have a job. But your medical condition may cause you to feel envious over less tangible things.

### MAKE THE BEST OF WHAT YOU HAVE

To get rid of this destructive emotion, concentrate on increasing those benefits and pleasures you *can* get out of life. Why worry about comparing yourself with somebody else? How is that going to help you? Sure, you may have diabetes. But that doesn't mean that you can't get a lot of enjoyment from life. Set up reasonable goals for yourself, considering what you *do* have and what you *can* do. Remember that you are who you are. Make the best of what your life has to offer.

## Loneliness

There is a difference between being alone and being lonely. Being alone simply means that there is no one else with you. This can be either good or bad. But being lonely is always negative. Loneliness is a sad, empty feeling in which you become upset by your awareness of being alone.

## WHY ARE YOU LONELY?

Why might you feel lonely? You may feel left out if you can't spend time with others the way you used to—because you're not feeling well, perhaps. Or you may feel lonely because you think that others don't understand your condition. You may simply feel different. And you may decide to change some of your relationships just because you're having a harder time dealing with people.

It's hard to be lonely—and not just because loneliness is such a bad feeling. You see, loneliness doesn't just happen. It actually takes effort to make and keep yourself lonely. There are many opportunities to enjoy the company of others. As a result, loneliness usually occurs out of choice rather than by accident. To be really lonely, you must purposely exclude everyone around you from your life. You have to always be on your guard, protecting yourself from the horrible possibility of making new friends!

## DO YOU *WANT* TO BE LONELY?

Why might you want to be lonely? There are four possible reasons. First, deep down you may actually enjoy being lonely. In fact, you may enjoy it so much that you refuse to do anything about it. Why? Because you may feel more comfortable when alone than when in the company of others.

Second, if you're lonely, you may be hard to please. You may feel that you don't want to even bother trying to create new relationships because no one meets all of your requirements.

Third, you may feel that you must be lonely. You may have resigned yourself to it. You may even tell yourself that this is an unavoidable part of having diabetes!

Fourth, and probably most important, you may be lonely because you're scared. You may be afraid of rejection. You may recall previous relationships that didn't work out the way you wanted, and feel that they are not worth the hurt and pain.

## END YOUR LONELY WAYS

Fortunately, whether your loneliness has been plaguing you for some time or is a relatively new problem, there is a light at the end of the tunnel! Recognize where your feeling of loneliness comes from. Admit to yourself that you should try to change this destructive emotion. Then do all you can to fight it.

### *Don't Be a Pusher*

The first step in ending loneliness is to stop pushing people away. It's likely that you're giving off unseen vibrations—vibrations that tell people you don't want them around. These vibrations can reduce your number of acquaintances, adding to your feeling of loneliness. This must stop. You have to learn to give off positive vibrations—the kind that welcome people instead of chasing them away. Smile at people. Show interest in what others have to say. Let them know that you like being with them.

### *Make Contact!*

Once you start giving off new, more positive vibes, you'll want to make more friends. How can you meet people? You can start by getting involved in an organization. Because you have diabetes, you may want to contact your local chapter of the American Diabetes Association or local diabetes support programs. There, you'll meet other people with similar concerns. Besides relieving your loneliness, the members of your support group may also share some valuable coping skills. You may even find ways of helping others.

If support groups aren't your cup of tea, try getting involved in a new learning activity or hobby. Take adult education courses, for example. This may help alleviate loneliness as well as boredom. Invite people to your home. (Be sure to pace yourself, though!) Most important, be as receptive as possible to the people that you meet. Try to see the good in everyone. Don't reject someone simply because there are a few things about them that you don't like.

You may feel that you'll have a harder time breaking free of loneliness if you are homebound. But even if you can't get out of the house, you still have connections to the outside world: your telephone and the Internet. If you're feeling particularly blue, your close friends and loved ones are just a phone call away. Remember, the special people in your life want you to be happy, and they'll be there to support you—even if "there" is at the other end of the telephone line.

If you own a computer, then you can get connected through the Internet. You'll soon find that your on-line resources are endless! You can meet people in on-line chat rooms who share your interests and concerns. You can even find support groups on the World Wide Web. Your doctor or diabetes educator may be able to give you some good resource sites on diabetes that can help you get started.

If you work at conquering loneliness, you'll feel much better about yourself and your life. This will make life more enjoyable, even with diabetes. Give yourself and others a chance, and your feelings of loneliness will disappear, regardless of the limitations your condition has placed on you.

## Putting It All Together

Living with any chronic medical problem can involve a number of painful emotions. But it is possible to cope with these emotions—to learn strategies that will eliminate or lessen them, and help you live more comfortably and happily. These strategies are just what the doctor—and family and friends—ordered!

# PART FOUR

# Interacting with Other People

# CHAPTER TWENTY-SIX

# Coping with Others—An Introduction

You do not live your life alone—unless you're reading this book on a deserted island in the South Pacific! You interact with many people every day. So you'll certainly want to be able to deal with any difficulties you are having in your interpersonal relationships. For example, you might be worried about what others are going to think now that you've been diagnosed with diabetes. How are they going to react? Are they going to ask questions? What kinds of answers will they listen to, and what answers will turn them away?

Obviously, different problems exist in different relationships. But before we begin discussing all the different people who may be part of your life, here are a few general guidelines you may find helpful.

## Do Unto Others . . .

When you interact with others, try not to get too wrapped up in your own feelings. If you disregard the feelings of those around you, you will also prevent them from getting close to you. So make a conscious effort to be considerate of others, just as you'd like them to be considerate of you.

What does this mean? Just this: *You're not the only one who has to cope with diabetes.* The important people in your life may also be having a hard time, simply because you mean a lot to them. Remember that. You might not realize that your problems affect those around you. You might think, "Why would they be upset? It's happening to me!" But if you give this some thought, you'll see that you're not being reasonable or fair.

Take your family, for example. A problem for you is also a problem for them. Of course, it may affect you in a different way. It's certainly true that you're the one who's experiencing the restrictions and the physical changes, as well as the apprehensions and anxieties. But your family doesn't like to see you suffer. You'll be better able to cope with these important people if you bear in mind that they are experiencing almost as much emotional turmoil as you are. In fact, this may explain why family members and friends might be unable to provide all of the support you want as quickly as you want it. Like you, they are probably going through a tough period of adjustment!

Then again, rather than being unaware of the emotions of others, you may feel guilty about the added burden you are placing on your family. This can be a hard feeling to cope with. Keep in mind, though, that you may be projecting this difficulty onto other people—and possibly adding to their problems in the process. Chances are, they don't feel as burdened as you may feel temporarily helpless or overwhelmed, and they will be eager to help.

## Change Yourself, Not Others

Do you feel that if you try hard enough, you'll be able to change the attitudes, feelings, or behaviors of others? Unfortunately, it doesn't work that way. Whether the people in your life accept your diabetes or deny that you have any problem at all, you won't be able to change them unless they want to change. So it makes sense to use your energy to change the one person over whom you do have control—yourself. Spend more time working on yourself, and less time worrying about others. In fact, once others see the changes in you, they may even alter their own attitudes. So help yourself. Be your own best friend.

## Look Through the Eyes of Others

If you have an argument with someone, you may believe that you're right and the other person is wrong. If this continues, nothing will be resolved, and the other person's behavior may drive you crazy because it seems so unreasonable.

Take a moment and look at the situation through the eyes of the other person. What might the other point of view be? Once you've done this, you'll be better able to explain how you feel in a way that he or she will understand. And then you'll be able to find a solution to almost any problem that might exist.

## Learn to Say "No"

Perhaps you've been feeling rotten, but others seem to want you to do more and more. In the past, you may have had trouble saying no—because either you felt guilty, or because you wanted to avoid disappointing the other person. But now things are a little different, and you really must curtail your generosity for the sake of your own well-being. Yes, this may give you the appearance of being selfish. But as long as you don't abuse it, this selfishness can be positive for you. Do for yourself; think of yourself. You're Number One, and that's the way it must be. Only if you take care of yourself will you be able to deal with others. The reverse does not necessarily hold true. If you always take care of others first, this may actually make you less able to care for yourself.

## Open the Lines of Communication

You'll find it far easier to deal with diabetes if you can rely on those closest to you, such as your partner, other family members, and close friends.

This social network can give you an added strength during the difficult period of adjustment to living with diabetes. But right now, you may find it difficult to even talk to others. So how can you possibly ask for their support? Well, your first job is to get the lines of communication open. The best way to get the conversation rolling is to be open and honest about the way you feel. If you say anything that upsets or hurts someone, you'll deal with it then. But first, get your feelings out on the table.

Perhaps you're waiting for others to approach you and offer their support. But since you're the one with diabetes, you may have to be the first person to talk about it. Some people may be reluctant to even mention the word in front of you. But if you bring it up and talk about it matter-of-factly, you may pave the way to more effective communication. Don't be ashamed to tell family and friends that you've been diagnosed with diabetes. It's a part of your life now. When others come to understand what you're experiencing, they will be better able to give you the support you need.

Joy, a forty-six-year-old mother of three, had recently been diagnosed with diabetes. She had already broken the news to her family, but was unsure how to approach the topic with her friends. She decided to let a few of her friends know about her diabetes at their weekly canasta game. As they sorted through their cards, Joy tentatively mentioned, "The doctor told me I have diabetes, and I have to be careful about what I eat." When she saw looks of concern on her friends' faces, she immediately added, "But don't worry—I'm looking forward to trying new recipes, and the doctor said I will have no problem beating you at canasta for many years to come!" The light tone of her comments reassured her friends. Joy helped her friends handle the news by showing them that she could handle it.

What if you're afraid to share your feelings? Certainly, fear can make communication difficult. For instance, if you're fearful that what you say may make the other person uncomfortable, you may hesitate to say it. Or perhaps it's their fear that's stopping you. Fortunately, there's an excellent solution to this problem. Simply reach out and physically touch the other person. By holding hands or sharing hugs, you can quickly bring about a type of sharing that doesn't require words. And in the process, you'll reestablish the lines of communication.

# Bring on the World

Now that we've introduced some general ideas, let's see how diabetes can affect the relationships that make up your life. Of course, not every chapter in this section will apply to you. You may choose to read only those that are appropriate, or you may decide to read all of them. However you choose to approach this material, you'll soon realize that problems exist in all relationships, but that you can learn to cope with them.

## CHAPTER TWENTY-SEVEN

# Your Family

Blood is thicker than water! Your family can be a critical factor in your successful adjustment to diabetes. Why? You're probably with your family more than you're with anyone else. If you get along well with members of your family, you have a ready source of emotional and practical support.

The impact of your diabetes on your family is sure to be profound. It seems that family members who are able to talk, share, cry, and hold on to each other during rough times have an easier time dealing with the problems posed by diabetes. On the other hand, when family members experience the impact but are unable to talk to one another about it, the adjustment is much more difficult. Which of these families sounds like yours? If your family is like most, it falls somewhere in between these two extremes.

Of course, different types of problems may pop up with different family members. So let's discuss how you can better deal with your partner, your children, and your parents.

## Living with Your Partner

Diabetes can certainly have an effect on your relationship. But this doesn't mean that your problems can't be resolved. There are very few problems that can't be resolved through better communication, understanding, and, if necessary, counseling. Let's discuss some of the ways in which diabetes may affect your relationship and various ways in which its impact can be lessened.

## CHANGES IN YOUR SOCIAL LIFE

Have restrictions caused by diabetes or related complications forced you to cut back on some of the social activities you used to enjoy with your partner? You might not be able to do as much now as you used to. This can be hard to take, especially if you and your partner had active social lives before the onset of your condition. Because your partner does not have diabetes, he or she may feel angry, frustrated, or helpless. You, on the other hand, may believe that your partner's social life has been put on hold, and it's all your fault. Or you may be angered by his or her seeming inability to accept these new restrictions.

Once you are able to manage your diabetes, you should be able to resume most of your activities. Until then, try to engage in activities that are not too challenging or strenuous. Sometimes, it's fun and relaxing just to watch a video with a few friends.

If your social life is still on hold even after your condition has stabilized, you'll have to ask yourself if this is due to fear, depression, or other emotional problems. If so, be sure to refer to the appropriate chapters earlier in this book.

## CHANGES IN FAMILY RESPONSIBILITIES

Diabetes may create the need for temporary or permanent changes in each family member's responsibilities, as your spouse and children take over some of the functions that you performed in the past. This can surely be a potential source of friction between you and your partner, especially if he or she receives a heavy share of the load.

How can you make changes as smoothly as possible, without causing your partner unnecessary distress? First, make the changes gradually. Try to avoid overwhelming your spouse—or other members of your family, for that matter. And be realistic in your expectations, keeping in mind that it takes time for *anyone* to comfortably incorporate new responsibilities into their routine.

How else can you help your spouse adjust to a heavier burden or responsibility? Make sure you leave some free time for the pleasures of life. It's only when new responsibilities seem to be all-consuming that serious problems occur. Be sure to look at any changes through the eyes of your partner. Consider how you'd feel if the situation were reversed. Think how upsetting it would be if you no longer had time for the things you enjoyed because of added responsibilities and pressures. Discuss the needed changes reasonably, and be gentle.

## IF YOUR PARTNER DENIES YOUR CONDITION

What can you do if your partner simply won't accept the fact that you have diabetes? You can, of course, try to "educate" your spouse, but do not go overboard. If you're constantly badgering you partner, pointing out how things must change because of your condition, it may only cause further denial. Keep in mind that your partner will not accept your condition until he or she is ready to do so. In the meantime, concentrate on improving your own thoughts and feelings. Others' feelings may change, but they will do so slowly, and probably not at your urgings.

## FINANCIAL PROBLEMS

Diabetes can present added money problems, especially if your spouse previously had little to do with family finances and must now share or take charge of financial responsibilities. But even if your partner has always taken part in the family's money matters, medical bills can make things tough. Both you and your spouse may worry whether all obligations can be met, and whether they will continue to be met over time.

What can you do? Sit down with your partner and talk over your financial problems. Try to be realistic and to reach practical solutions. Admit that new problems may arise, but emphasize the fact that these frequently have a way of working themselves out. If not, you will deal with them as they develop. Be patient, be communicative, and—above all—be positive. (For tips on dealing with financial problems, see chapter 17.)

## HAS YOUR SEX LIFE BEEN AFFECTED?

Diabetes can affect sexual relations. If this is a problem for you and your partner, or if you'd just like to learn more about the possible impact that diabetes can have on sex, see chapter 31. There, you'll learn how sexual problems can be worked out so that sex can remain an important and pleasurable part of your life.

## IN SICKNESS AND IN HEALTH? SORRY!

Unfortunately, some relationships have ended because of chronic medical problems. Diabetes-related fears, symptoms, and side effects certainly have the potential to drive a wedge into what may have previously been a good relationship, replacing feelings of closeness and intimacy with coldness and distance. This can wash the "magic" right out of a relationship.

What should you do if your spouse is frightened and "wants out"? First, be aware that any problems may not be entirely your partner's fault. For instance, you may be too apprehensive to enjoy your relationship, and your and your spouse's combined problems may be creating a horrible package of anxiety, depression, hopelessness, and panic. What should you do after you try to view the problem objectively? Get help. This package isn't one that you can—or should—handle alone. If communication has become a problem in your house, you may not be able to talk to your partner. The aid of a professional or an objective outsider may help to resolve some of the problems that you and your partner have been unable to work out yourselves. If your partner doesn't seem open to outside help, get some counseling for yourself. Regardless of the results of your efforts to save your relationship, any support you can muster will only improve your emotional well-being.

### A MARITAL (CON)SUMMATION

Every relationship has its ups and downs, with problems that have to be worked out. Of course, diabetes does make relationships more vulnerable to crises and arguments. But by giving added attention to your partner's feelings and needs, you will find that many—if not all—of these problems can be worked out over time. And isn't your relationship worth the added effort? Once problem spots have been smoothed out, your spouse may become your greatest ally in dealing with your condition.

## Dealing with Your Children

Children—regardless of how old they are!—may be especially vulnerable to the stresses and fears that occur when a family member has a chronic illness. Certainly, at this time you may not be able to help them as much as you used to, or to spend as much time with them as you'd like. But you can surely use the time you do spend with them as productively as possible, and you can also help your children to handle any fears or changes that may be bothering them. How? Let's see how you can help you children better cope with your condition.

### ENCOURAGE QUESTIONS

When you talk to your children, make sure that you take the time to answer any questions they may have. Discussions, if handled properly, will not only be helpful for your children, but can also provide both you and your kids with a special feeling of closeness.

But what if your kids don't ask questions? Remember that if your children really don't want to, they won't, no matter how much encouragement you give them. But you should let them know that they can ask anything they want. Remember, fears and anxieties can be very destructive if they're kept bottled up inside. Once your children know that they have the option of talking to you freely, they can decide what they wish to discuss.

How should you answer your children's questions? This depends on the ages of your kids, as well as on how detailed an answer they're looking for. The best advice is to provide direct answers to their questions. Don't go into detail unless your children ask for more information. Try to determine exactly what they want to know. This may be tricky, as even your children may not know what answers they're looking for. So just start talking, and provide them with more information as they ask for it.

Certainly, whenever you're speaking to your children about illness—especially if your kids are young—you should be careful not to frighten them. Remember that children have great imaginations, and often blow things out of proportion. You do want your kids to continue talking to you about your condition. If you show that you accept diabetes and that you welcome questions about it, this will greatly benefit your relationship with them.

If you have difficulty discussing your illness with your children, it might be a good idea to speak to a professional—your doctor, their pediatrician, a psychologist, or a social worker—and have him or her take control of the discussion.

## FOCUS ON QUALITY, NOT QUANTITY

As you adjust to living with diabetes, there may be times when you can't spend as much time with your children as you would like to. If you develop a diabetes-related complication, you may be prevented from doing a lot of what you'd like to do. How can you solve this dilemma? Honestly explain to your children that, at times, you'll want to rest, and you may not be able to participate in the usual family routine. Then come to an agreement with them when you're feeling better. This arrangement will show your children that you're aware of their unhappiness, and that you do want to spend more time with them

Also, try to be less concerned with *quantity time*—the number of minutes and hours you spend with your kids—and more concerned with *quality time*—special time during which you share feelings and pleasurable activities. If your time together is well spent, with plenty of talking and laughing, you'll make up for any missed time. And as you share your thoughts with your children, you'll be helping them to better handle your medical condition.

## ADOLESCENTS

During adolescence, children begin to assert their independence. Look out, world, the future generation is coming! Adolescents want to start moving away from the family setting and its responsibilities. Even under normal circumstances, this creates problems in many homes. Add a parent with diabetes to the picture, and the problem is compounded. Why? If you develop complications, your teen may have to help out more than usual around the house. At the same time, he or she probably wants to do less around the house, and be away more. How can you cope with this predicament? Well, in truth, you may not be able to change your teen much. But perhaps you can learn to cope in a way that, at the very least, keeps you sane! Let's learn more about dealing with teens.

### *Don't Expect Miracles!*

First, realize that dealing with teens is quite different from dealing with younger kids—which you probably already know. As already discussed, teens are far more absorbed in themselves than in their families. Remember that they are going through quite a few difficult adjustments of their own. Of course, not all teens are alike. Some are less self-centered and more sensitive and compassionate than others. Certainly, you know your child better than anyone. But perhaps you now expect your usually insensitive child to rise to the occasion and enthusiastically pitch in with household chores. Be aware that you are probably setting yourself up for disappointment if you expect your child to change so significantly.

Of course, this doesn't mean that you shouldn't discuss your condition with your teen. Talk to your child candidly, treating him or her like an adult. This will probably provide the best chance for a positive response. Think about the concerns your adolescent might have regarding your diabetes, and try to be reassuring. If your child feels comfortable talking to you about your condition, encourage discussion. But you should respect your child's wishes if he or she does not wish to talk about your illness.

### *When You Need Your Teen to Pitch In*

Because of your condition, your adolescent may now have to shoulder more responsibilities. But will your teen be willing to help out? That's the real question!

Seventeen-year-old Laurie felt guilty about not helping out more at home. However, she thought that giving in would be a sign of weakness. (Heaven forbid!) This caused Laurie a lot of anguish—which, of course she didn't want to discuss with her parents. Because of the guilt she was experiencing, Laurie escaped by spending even more time than usual out of the house—and less time helping out! Laurie's parents sat her down, and together they worked out a compromise. Laurie would not have to spend all her time helping out at home, but she would make herself available when necessary. After reaching an agreement, both Laurie and her parents felt closer to one another—and Laurie felt a good deal better about herself.

As you can see, it may pay to take the initiative and offer a reasonable compromise. Just showing that you understand your teen's feelings may help. Perhaps things won't seem so hopeless to your child, after all.

Another tactic, too, may prove helpful. If your adolescent must take on some adult chores, consider that he or she may also be ready to enjoy a few adult privileges and pleasures—within reason of course. Adolescents will usually be more willing to help out if they know that they will be treated and trusted in a more grown-up way.

Remember that you can go only so far in trying to get your adolescent's cooperation. You can't move mountains. Continue to be as constructive as you can, putting as little pressure on your child as possible in order to keep the door open to good relations. As long as you know you've tried, you can hold your head up high.

## Dealing with Your Parents

Parents often have difficulty coping with a child's illness—even if their "child" is an adult. Therefore, anticipate that your parents will have a rough time. This, of course, will make coping harder for you, too. Why?

You don't want your parents to suffer. And you know how your parents feel, because you'd certainly be upset if your child were ill.

If your relationship with your parents is good, then you're among the lucky ones. But what if you normally have difficulty dealing with your parents? Having diabetes won't help! Regardless of the type of relationship you've had previously, consider how your parents have treated you since your diagnosis. Have they ignored or minimized your condition? Or have they smothered you? Let's look at these two possible reactions, and see how you can better cope with your parents.

## THE IGNORERS

Parents who ignore or play down your diabetes often do so because they can't deal with it. They can't face the fact that their child is sick. Worse, many parents agonize over the possibility that your problem might have something to do with them. While this may not make any sense to you, your parents may be afraid that they did something to contribute to your illness, or that you inherited the condition from them. To avoid these intolerable thoughts, they may try to deny that you have diabetes, or they may minimize your illness, hoping it will go away.

Remember what I said in the previous chapter about seeing a situation through someone else's eyes? Don't you think that it holds true in this case? As you look through the eyes of your seemingly indifferent parents, you'll probably realize that this is the only way in which they can cope with the situation right now. Yes, their behavior may change over time, but the change will be gradual and not necessarily in response to your urgings.

## THE SMOTHERERS

Parents who smother believe that if you have any kind of problem, they must take care of you. Having diabetes certainly fits this requirement. It doesn't matter what your marital status is or how old you are. What matters to them is that they are your parents—they feel responsible for your welfare. They'll call frequently, asking how you're doing. They'll want to know what they can do to help. They may come over as often as possible to make sure that you're okay. Whether they visit or not, they'll constantly bombard you with questions about your health and activities.

What can you do, short of moving out of town and taking on a new identity? Again, look at yourself—and your condition—through the eyes of your parents. How do you think they feel? They care about you. What do they see? They see a child who needs them! You may not agree with them, but understanding their point of view should help you better communicate with them and more effectively explain how you feel.

## WHAT IF TALKING DOESN'T HELP?

If you've talked to your parents and haven't succeeded in modifying their behavior, at least you know you've tried. This alone may help you feel better! What else can you do? Concentrate on helping yourself feel better. If your parents are unhappy with you because you seem to be rejecting their well-meaning intentions, so be it. If they are unhappy with you because you're making it hard for them to ignore your condition, that's fine, too.

By the way, if you're unhappy with parents who are ignorers, you'd probably love them to smother you for a while. And if you don't like smothering parents, the thought of being left alone is probably very appealing. There's rarely a perfect situation or relationship, and no one gets along with everyone all the time. So instead of complaining about your parents' faults, try to look at the positives in their behavior. This may make you feel better, and will certainly help you avoid going crazy over their actions.

## HOW MUCH SHOULD YOU TELL YOUR PARENTS?

A common question of people with chronic illnesses concerns how much they should tell their parents about their problem. Have you worried about this, too? First, think about your parents. How do they usually deal with unpleasant situations? Then ask yourself what you want to share with them. Next imagine how they would react to this, and how you would handle their reactions. All these factors will help you decide how much you should tell them.

For instance, you might wish you could share your fears and worries with your parents because of the reassurances it would bring. It would certainly be nice to know that you don't have to face something unpleasant alone. But what if your parents couldn't readily accept your problems even if they wanted to? It might be more detrimental to tell them things that they couldn't handle. So don't impulsively blurt your feelings out. By spending a little time figuring out what's best, you can help yourself feel a lot better. You'll probably improve your relationship with your parents, as well.

Finally, keep in mind that it's sometimes easier to talk to one parent than to the other. Consider telling one parent what's bothering you, and letting that parent tell the other. For example, your mother may be able to get through to your father better than you can. This will make things easier for everybody.

## A Familial Finale

As you learn to cope with diabetes, you're biggest ally—and an important source of emotional support and practical assistance—may be your family. By learning to deal with your family members in the best possible way, you'll not only make things easier for them, but also make them better able to help you cope with diabetes.

## CHAPTER TWENTY-EIGHT

# Friends and Colleagues

Aside from family, you also deal with friends and colleagues on a daily or near daily basis. Are there any ways in which you can better deal with these important people? Of course!

## Dealing with Your Friends

Before your diagnosis, your relationships with your friends may have been fairly effortless. Unfortunately, diabetes can change that. You may be surprised or hurt by the seeming aloofness of some friends, while others may be too supportive. Then, of course, there are the special problems that may crop up because of your condition, such as the need to ask for help. These problems can sometimes take a toll on seemingly strong friendships. How can you handle this? Read on!

### BE PREPARED FOR DIFFERENT REACTIONS

How have your friends reacted to your diabetes? How many even know what diabetes is all about? They may have read about it, and at first they may have thought they understood it. But because they haven't been directly affected by it, they may not be able to really understand what you are experiencing. Some may want to learn more; some may want to forget what little they already know.

Certainly you should be prepared for a variety of reactions to your condition. Some friends, for instance, may seem uninterested and distant. Why would a friend seem distant at a time when you need special support? Well, some people may not know what to say to you. What should they ask you? How should they talk to you? Should they even mention your condition? They may not want to run the risk of stirring up unpleasant feelings for you—or for themselves, if they don't know how to respond. Their doubts and fears may cause so much tension that they don't even want to be with you. Of course, some friends may be very supportive—perhaps *too* supportive! There may be times when friends keep asking you how you are, or offering help, when you'd rather be left alone.

Certainly, friendships can be hurt because of misunderstandings and uncertainties. Can anything be done to prevent these problems from undermining your friendships, or do you have to be a hermit for the rest of your life? Don't despair. There are things you can do to improve the situation.

Try to establish ground rules with your friends. If you're the kind of person who likes to be asked how you feel, let your friends know. If you'd rather not be asked, let your friends know that, too. If your preferences fluctuate (sometimes feeling talkative about your condition, but at other times reluctant to even think about it), let your friends know. Your changing feelings may be harder for friends to deal with, so let them know that they can talk to you whenever they really want to. You'll let them know if and when you're having trouble.

Clear up the question marks. If you tell your friends how you feel and what your needs and desires are, fewer unknowns will exist. The uneasiness about what to do or say, which can hurt friendships, will be reduced. Your friends will become more aware of your needs, and will feel closer to you and less afraid.

## CHANGING PLANS

Don't you love having to change plans with a friend at the last minute? Probably not. So you can understand how your friends might feel about it. But as you learn to cope with diabetes—or if you must cope with a complication—there will most likely be times when you don't feel up to going out, or when some aspect of your treatment must take precedence over your social activities. Good friends, who understand or at least try to understand what you're going through, will probably be able to accept these last-minute cancellations. Others may not hide their annoyance when you have to cancel plans.

So how can you remedy this situation? It's a good idea to sit down with some of your closest friends and work out a solution to the problem. You can even ask them for suggestions. Although you may not always get the understanding you want, you'll probably find at least one or two friends who will be willing to work on a solution to any problems you may have.

## ASKING FOR HELP

As you learn to live with diabetes, you may have a greater need to call on your friends for help. Are you becoming more selfish? No—although it may seem that way to you. You'd probably like to be able to function completely independently, but it just may not be possible. The reality is that there are certain things that must be taken care of, and if you can't take care of them yourself, you must ask others to help you. So if you need help, reach out for it. That's better than pushing yourself too hard and suffering the consequences.

When planning to ask for help, keep in mind that older friendships tend to be stronger and more resilient. Longtime friends will probably be more receptive when approached for favors. Newer or more casual friends should probably not be burdened as much. Without giving a friendship a chance to become firmly planted on your hook, you may lose your prize fish—a good, long-lasting friendship. Also, base your choice on the type of help you need. Aim for a proper fit. (By the way, no matter how old and dear the friend, once you feel up to it, it would be nice to show your appreciation with an unexpected gift or gesture.)

What should you do if your friends complain or show resentment when you request help? Back off for a while. In addition, try to talk it over with them. Discuss these problems when the conflict can still be resolved; don't let them build up until the friendship is destroyed. If your efforts to mend the friendship fail, remember this: Friends who can't understand your need for help are not very good friends anyway.

## LOSING FRIENDS

What if the people you thought were your friends don't call or visit? What if they seem reluctant to make any plans with you, preferring to "wait and see how you feel"? When friends seem to drift away, it's certainly sad. But remember that it was not your decision to end the friendship. And you don't want it to be your problem!

Why might this have happened? Maybe your friend felt uncomfortable being with you. Maybe he or she was "turned off" by the fact that you have a medical problem, or felt unsure of what to say or do. Whatever the reason, you've probably learned a hard, unpleasant lesson: You can't change someone else's feelings.

If a friend, or anyone else, cannot handle your condition, you may feel rejected. This can be devastating—especially if you fear that you won't be able to develop any other meaningful relationships! This is not true. You are the same person you were before your diagnosis. Keep telling yourself this so that you can restore any confidence that may have been shaken by your friend's action. Be reassured that most people who lose friends do make new ones. Anyway, you don't really want a "friend" who is uncomfortable around you. You want a friend who likes you for who you are—diabetes and all! And there are plenty of wonderful, understanding people out there. So don't give up!

# Dealing with Your Colleagues

If you work, you're probably spending many hours a week with a number of colleagues. These people are likely to show a variety of reactions to your condition (if they know about it), as well as to any impact your condition may have on your work. Let's discuss some of the ways in which you may better cope with your colleagues.

## SHOULD YOU TELL YOUR COLLEAGUES?

Hopefully, if you're comfortable with yourself, others will be, too. Many colleagues will take your condition in stride, and won't even think about it. Might it be helpful to provide them with some basic information on diabetes? It could be, although you should realize that this will not necessarily improve their attitude toward you or your condition. Unfortunately, knowledge doesn't always lead to understanding. However, just knowing that you've tried to help your colleagues understand might make you feel better.

While you may be tempted not to even bother telling your coworkers about your condition, remember that one or two colleagues should be aware that you have diabetes, and should know how to help you in case of an emergency.

## WHEN COLLEAGUES ARE RESENTFUL

Once you have mastered diabetes management, there's no reason why you shouldn't be able to stick to your regular work schedule. However, if your diabetes is poorly controlled, or if you have developed a diabetes-related complication, you may need to reduce your work hours. This plan may not be accepted graciously by your fellow workers and may cause bitterness and strain among your working relationships.

If you have to curtail your working hours, or find that you must miss work frequently, you may encounter some resentment. As discussed above, at this point you may decide to explain your situation to your colleagues. But accept the fact that some people just won't want to understand what's happening to you and why. Remember: You can't change somebody else. If a colleague—or anybody else, for that matter—can't handle or understand what's going on, that's his or her problem. You can try to educate people about diabetes, but you shouldn't make their attitude your problem. If you've got an employer with an open mind, you're way ahead of the game. Don't be as concerned about the attitudes of coworkers. Instead, concentrate on doing what's best for you.

## Time to Punch Out

Whether you're dealing with friends or coworkers, always take one day at a time. Don't worry about problems that have not occurred yet and, for that matter, may never occur. If your diabetes does cause a problem, be precise in identifying exactly what the problem is. Then don't hesitate to employ the best strategies you know to resolve the dilemma, and to restore good relations between you and the people you deal with in your day-to-day life.

# CHAPTER TWENTY-NINE

# Your Physician

How do you feel about your physician? (What a question!) Some people see physicians as gods. Others feel that they're cold professionals who don't really want to help. Your own view of your doctor will help determine how your treatment progresses. You may find that your feelings toward your physician—or toward physicians in general—have changed since your diagnosis. Some people with diabetes don't have much confidence in their physicians, probably because they haven't been "cured." Others recognize that they should not expect miracles, and continue to rely on their doctors to offer the best treatment possible.

This chapter focuses on the importance of a good doctor–patient relationship, and shows you how you can improve your dealings with your own physician. Remember that the suggestions offered here can be applied to your relationship with any member of your treatment team. Your treatment team is made up of a number of professionals who are all working together toward a common goal—to help you. You want to best utilize their professional services, don't you?

# Creating a Good Doctor–Patient Relationship

Your doctor must be someone in whom you have confidence medically. The reason for this is clear. But, just as important, you'll want someone with whom you're comfortable personally. The more comfortable you are with your physician, the more likely you'll comply with the prescribed treatment. And, of course, you must remember that you'll have to see your physician a good deal more often than someone without a chronic medical problem.

A great many factors will determine your ability to feel comfortable with your physician, including your personality, your doctor's personality, your doctor's philosophy regarding treatment, and more. Remember that the chemistry between a doctor and each patient is unique. A physician who is "perfect" for someone else may not be right for you. You'll have to pick somebody whom *you* feel good about, so your relationship gets off to a good start and continues on track.

## SET COMMUNICATION GROUND RULES

It's vital to set communication ground rules with your doctor. Because diabetes requires a great deal of self-care, you'll want to get all the facts. However much information you want, be sure to make your needs clear to your doctor. Be aware that there's nothing wrong with saying something like, "Doctor, I really want all the information about my condition. But please remember that I'm very sensitive, so try to break it to me as gently as possible!"

## ASK QUESTIONS

You are certainly well within your rights to question any aspect of the treatment that is prescribed for you. Some people, of course, prefer not to ask questions, but to simply follow the directions of their physician. This is also within your rights. Remember that you want to do everything possible to help youself, so the more you know, the better.

Of course, we all want to have confidence in our doctors—to believe that they know what they're talking about. This doesn't mean, however, that you must blindly accept everything your doctor says. For the most part, physicians respect patients who ask questions. Don't feel that if you disagree, your physician will throw you out. If you are unsure about a recommendation, question it.

## Getting the Most from Office Visits

Most of our communications with doctors takes place during office visits. We certainly want these visits to be as helpful and productive as possible. But as you may know, this is sometimes more easily said than done. All of us have come home from a doctor's visit and realized that we forgot to ask an important question. Or perhaps we did ask the question, and then promptly forgot the answer! Nothing can be more frustrating—especially since it is often so difficult to reach a doctor by phone! Fortunately, there are ways in which you can avoid this frustration. Let's look at some of the easy things you can do to get the most from your office visits.

### MAKING A LIST

Before each appointment, it's important to prepare a list of all the questions you want to ask the doctor. Don't wait until the night before your office visit to put your list together. Instead, prepare the list by jotting down notes whenever a question or piece of information pops into your mind.

Although making a list may seem elementary, it is an excellent way to obtain the information you need to understand your condition, properly take care of yourself, and guide your treatment. Don't be concerned that the doctor won't like your preparing a list of questions. Most good doctors do appreciate this practice because it tends to structure the appointments more efficiently. However, if your doctor doesn't like it, ask yourself this: Whose treatment and condition is on the line, anyway?

Many people worry that the questions they wish to ask are too trivial, or even foolish. Remember that the only foolish question is the unasked one! If you need further explanation about your treatment, feel free to ask and be as straightforward as possible. This will make it easier for your doctor to respond with the information you need.

## GETTING THE ANSWERS

As your doctor answers your questions, be sure to listen carefully. How annoying is it to realize that you've been looking at the next question, rather than listening to the doctor's response?! If you're worried that you won't remember everything that goes on in your doctor's office, there are three ways in which you can aid your memory. The first is to jot down notes as each question is answered. The second is to bring a tape recorder. The third is to bring a family member or close friend.

It can be very helpful to go to the doctor with somebody, because two sets of ears are always better than one. It's easy to miss what's being said because of the tension you may feel in the doctor's office. Having an extra listener will increase the likelihood that all important information will be retained. This will also take some of the pressure off you, helping you to relax and more efficiently listen and respond. Following the doctor's visit, you and your companion will be able to sit down and compare notes about what was said.

If you do decide to bring a family member or friend with you, make sure that this person knows what you want to accomplish during the appointment. Discuss in advance the kinds of questions you want to ask, and the information you hope to obtain. Your family member will then be able to jump in and ask any questions that he or she feels you've overlooked.

It's also important to speak up when you don't understand your doctor's answers because they're either too vague or technical. Don't hesitate to question your doctor further. Perhaps he or she is used to discussing cases with other doctors, and has become accustomed to using specialized, scientific terms. Perhaps other patients have been too intimidated to ask for clarifications! Whatever the reason, don't be afraid to speak up. And don't be embarrassed. Your goal is to talk more comfortably and intelligently about what's happening to you. If you don't understand what's going on or if you don't agree with a treatment plan, let your doctor know.

## Getting Second Opinions

If you disagree with your physician, you may want to get a second opinion. You should always get a second opinion before major surgery (unless it's an emergency procedure). However, many people are worried about hurting their physician's feelings. Don't let that stop you. Think logically. Most physicians will accept your desire to get a second opinion. It will either confirm what they feel or point out the need for further discussion. If your physician objects to your getting a second opinion, you should certainly ask why. This does not mean that you should make a habit of going for second opinions. Nor should you continually shop around for the "ideal" physician. No such person exists.

## Being Able to Reach Your Physician

Do you know what's really frustrating? How about when you call your physician and have to wait hours before your call is returned? This may be one of your criteria when searching for a physician. Make sure you feel confident that your physician will promptly return your calls.

After you've lived with diabetes for a while, you'll know when you should call and when it's not necessary. Certain symptoms, such as those of hypoglycemia or DKA, may require you to immediately contact your physician. Other symptoms, such as minor aches and pains, or minor blood glucose level fluctuations, may not have to be reported immediately. Discuss this with your physician. Find out how he or she would feel if you were to call when you were having problems. Ask about the kind of things that should be phoned in. Also ask when would be the best times to call.

## You're Not "Locked In"

Some people are reluctant to change physicians. Others seem to change physicians more often than they change their socks! If you're not happy with your physician, you're not under any obligation to continue to see him or her. Don't continue to visit a particular physician if you feel you can't ask questions, if you feel intimidated, or if you feel that you can't call when there's a problem. Don't stick with your physician if you don't have confidence in the information you're being given, or in the course of treatment that's being prescribed. Finally, don't continue seeing your physician if you feel that he or she doesn't care about you or doesn't have your best interests at heart.

However, before you start looking for another doctor, carefully examine *why* you want to switch. Are you changing because your doctor doesn't give you the appropriate information at the appropriate time? Are you changing because your doctor doesn't seem compassionate enough? Try to pinpoint the cause of the problem.

After you determine what you don't like about your doctor, attempt to decide if your grievance is valid. Be aware that virtually any person who is diagnosed with diabetes will experience anxiety—anxiety that can spill over into the doctor-patient relationship, causing problems. Physicians may not always have the answers. Thus tensions may rise even higher. Is this tension affecting your judgment of your doctor? Or is there, in fact, a real problem that must be dealt with?

If the problem is valid, you have three options. Your first option is to continue seeing your doctor under the present (miserable) conditions. Your second option is to be more assertive, and to discuss the situation with your doctor in the hopes of improving your relationship. Your third option is to simply change doctors without trying to salvage the relationship.

Obviously, your first option is not a good one. Staying with a doctor who makes you miserable is not going to contribute to your well-being.

The second option, however, is worth considering. Many people find that if they talk to their doctor about their concerns in a constructive, positive way, problems can be ironed out. When this is possible, it is sometimes unnecessary to change doctors. How might you go about approaching your doctor concerning problems in your relationship? Don't try to accomplish this over the telephone or at the tail end of a regular examination. Instead, set up a separate consultation so that you will have the time to sit down and discuss your concerns. Once your doctor is made aware of the problem, you may very well be able to reach a mutually satisfactory solution.

But perhaps you don't feel comfortable approaching your doctor in this way. If you are afraid of being honest—or feel that your doctor simply can't provide you with the care you need—this relationship may not be the one for you. If so, your third option may be your best choice.

## Just What the Doctor Ordered

Your goal in life may not have been to become as knowledgeable as possible regarding diabetes. Nor is it likely that your goal was to keep ongoing records of your medical history, or to sharpen your communication skills. But you'll find that your efforts will pay big dividends when dealing with doctors—the biggest dividends being greater health and an improved ability to cope with diabetes.

# CHAPTER THIRTY

# Comments from Others

As Ralph Kramden of *The Honeymooners* would say, "Some people have a BIG MOUTH!" You may agree with this when you think of some of the comments made by the people around you. They may be close friends or even relatives, but that doesn't mean they know how to talk to you about your condition. They may say things that they think are true, witty, intelligent, or even sympathetic. But you may think otherwise! There may be times when a comment makes you want to implant your knuckles into the speaker's teeth! Or a comment might make you wonder if you're talking to a graduate of the Ignoramus School of Tactlessness.

As you now know, you cannot change other people. You cannot make them more sensitive or teach them how to be more tactful. But you can learn to cope with some of the ridiculous comments you hear.

You're probably now eager to learn a few coping strategies. But before we discuss the techniques that will help you cope with annoying comments—and the annoying people who make them—it's important to realize that most people say things out of sincere concern. They may be trying to make you feel better, to show their support, or to show an interest in you by questioning how you're feeling. Despite the good intentions behind these comments, though, it may not always be possible to respond to them politely and thoughtfully. The problem is that hearing the same questions over and over can get on your nerves. Initially, you may try to gently respond to comments and questions, or to politely change the subject. But this may not always work.

Certainly, some people with diabetes avoid unwelcome comments simply by keeping their condition a secret. For the purpose of this chapter, though, let's assume that we're discussing those comments that you can't avoid, made by people who haven't yet learned to tune into your feelings. If you've never experienced any comments of this nature, that's great! But read on anyway. You never know when a tip might come in handy!

## How Should You Respond?

Many of the things that people say to you may be legitimate comments but may bug you just the same. Other remarks may be made without any consideration of your feelings. But it doesn't matter why a comment is inappropriate. What's important is that you handle these comments in a way that makes you feel comfortable.

How might you respond to an annoying comment? There are three ways of responding that might work—that is, that might prevent a further stream of remarks, while making you as comfortable as possible. The first way is to ignore the comment. This is not always easy, especially if the person persistently waits for your answer or seems genuinely insulted by your lack of response. But if you are able to change the subject or walk away, you may get that person to stop asking questions.

The second way of responding to comments is to answer in a rational and intelligent way, explaining how you feel or what you sincerely want to communicate to the other person. This may satisfy the person so that he stops making remarks or asking questions. But, of course, there's a limit to the number of times you can explain something, especially if what you're trying to say isn't being understood or accepted. (And this certainly isn't good for your physical health!)

As you see, you may not always be able to cope by ignoring a remark or responding to it rationally. So what can you do when these two approaches fail? You can respond humorously. Why would this work? Well, the person's comment is really unanswerable. So you're going to have a little fun with your response, and humorously let that person know that his remark may have been somewhat inappropriate. This technique is called *paradoxical intention.* Let's use the remainder of the chapter to look at some of the comments you may hear, and see how you can use paradoxical intention to answer the unanswerable—without losing your sanity or saying things that you might later regret.

## "You Look Awful!"

It can be very upsetting when somebody says, "Wow, you look lousy!" You may feel lousy, but you certainly don't want to be reminded of it. You surely don't want to think that the way you feel is so obvious to others. You'd like to believe that you at least look okay to those around you. Even if it's said sympathetically, this remark may be insulting. So what can you say? You might respond, "Thank you, so do you!" or "Good! All my hard work has paid off." Or if you're really in a cynical mood, you might say, "I know I look lousy. That comes from hearing people tell me I look lousy all the time!" Of course, you could always say, "That makes sense, since I don't feel so hot, either!"

## "How Can You Stand Giving Yourself Injections?"

In response to this profoundly sympathetic expression of curiosity, you might want to say, "It's really not a problem. Let me give you one so you can see how much fun it is!" Or you might want to point out other feelings, such as, "I've grown rather accustomed to being able to live!" Or you might simply say, "I don't stand it. I usually sit down when I do it!" People will get the message. You may not like this aspect of diabetes, but at least you're learning to cope with it.

## "What Is Diabetes?"

Some people really don't understand what diabetes is all about. (Really!) So they'll bluntly ask you to explain your condition. This kind of question usually does show genuine concern, so under some circumstances you might want to simply explain a little more about what diabetes is and how it affects you. But if this is the twenty-fourth time you've heard the same question, it may be hard to respond calmly. What could you say that would not be unnecessarily cruel, but would still allow you to feel better about the way you handled the situation—and hopefully end the question-and-answer session? How about, "Let's forget you even brought it up. Then can you keep your streak going?" Or how about, "I don't know anything about it either. How's the weather?" This is not meant to suggest that you should be unfeeling in your answers. However, if you need to let the speaker know that you don't appreciate these questions, this'll do it!

## Other Lovable Comments

What are some of the other comments that you may hear? How many of these have come your way? "Is diabetes contagious?" "Why don't you quit your job?" "Are you sure you still need insulin?" "Do you feel like a pincushion?" "Rest. Don't do anything!" "What is the prognosis?" "Do you miss sugar?" "Wow, have you changed!" "You must miss the way you used to feel." "I sure don't envy you!" "If you ate right, you'd feel better!"

It would fill volumes to include all of the comments that you might hear from "well-meaning" friends or relatives. Hopefully, by reading the previous examples, you've gotten a good idea of how you can respond in a humorous way. Perhaps you'll be able to come up with some additional goodies. Remember that you don't necessarily want to be sarcastic or cruel. Rather, you want to show the speaker that you're feeling well enough to respond with humor and spirit. And you want to show that you can certainly do without this person's "helpful" bits of information and "words of encouragement"!

Perhaps you're thinking, "I could never say those things. It's just not my style." Well, you don't always have to. But you can at least think these comments. Even that may help you feel better! And keep in mind that even if you don't want to use this type of response all the time, you may want to use it occasionally—when it seems appropriate for you. As you learn to respond more comfortably to these comments, you'll find that you can handle them more calmly. Then you'll be able to minimize the sarcasm, and respond with more humorous and enjoyable answers.

## The Last Word

One of the most common and yet most irritating comments has been saved for last. Imagine somebody who is supposedly sympathetic turning to you with eyes full of compassion and concern, saying, "I heard of someone who died from diabetes!" As you turn to walk away, you respond, "I heard of someone who died for telling someone with diabetes what you just told me!" You walk away, head held high and a smile on your face, leaving the astonished well-wisher behind you.

# CHAPTER THIRTY-ONE

# Sex and Diabetes

This chapter is not rated *R* for Restricted. Rather, it is rated *E* for Essential. Why? If you are sexually active, you certainly don't want diabetes to prevent you from having an enjoyable sex life.

Has diabetes decreased your sexual appetite? Certainly, some people with diabetes experience a decreased interest in sex. As a matter of fact, decreased sexual interest is quite common with a number of chronic medical problems. What kind of sexual relationship did you have before you were diagnosed? If you had a good one, you may have an easier time getting over any obstacles that diabetes may have thrown into your path. If your sexual relationship wasn't good, it is unlikely that having diabetes will make it better! You may need some professional help to keep things from breaking down altogether. And if complications have created problems, alterations may have to be made. But hope is not lost. If you unite with your partner to work things out together, reassure each other, relearn how to please each other, and show a desire for each other, in all likelihood, you will eventually resume enjoyable sexual relations.

Sexual problems related to diabetes can be physiological or psychological in origin, or they may be a combination of the two. Let's look at both types of causes, and at possible means of coping with sexual problems.

# Physical Problems

Can physical problems alter your sexual relations? Yes. Depending on the degree to which diabetes and its treatment is affecting you, and depending on your previous level of sexual interest and activity, physical problems may either alter sexual desire or make it more difficult to engage in sexual relations. Let's learn a little about these possibilities.

## PROBLEMS SPECIFIC TO MEN

Any man would almost certainly shudder at the thought that he might experience erectile dysfunction, commonly known as impotence. Unfortunately, this is the most common sexual problem associated with diabetes in men.

It's probably safe to say that for some men, the possibility of impotence is one of the most frightening aspects of diabetes. So, before we begin our discussion, you should know that erectile dysfunction is *not* inevitable. And today, several safe, effective treatments are available to help correct the problem.

### *Erectile Dysfunction*

Men with sexual problems related to diabetes may have trouble achieving or sustaining an erection even though they have a normal sex drive. While medical experts agree that this problem is due to complications of diabetes, there is still some debate over the primary cause. Some doctors argue that nerve damage (neuropathy) impairs a man's ability to respond to sexual stimulation. Others believe that damange to the circulatory system (cardiovascular disease) interferes with blood flow to the penis. Without adequate blood flow to fill the spongy tissue of the penis, a man cannot achieve an erection.

Whether the cause of erectile dysfunction is neuropathy or cardiovascular disease, the root of the problem is almost always poor blood glucose control. That's where tight control comes into play. Research has conclusively proven that as diabetes management improves, the risk of neuropathy and cardiovascular disease decreases substantially—along with the risk of erection impairment. Other diabetes-related risk factors for impotence include the duration of diabetes, obesity, the presence of other diabetic complications, and the use of blood pressure medications.

***What to Do About Impotence.*** There are a number of treatment options available today to treat erectile dysfunction. The latest pharmaceutical offered for the treatment of impotence is sildenafil (Viagra). This drug relaxes blood vessels in the penis, allowing more blood to flow into it to create an erection. Sildenafil requires sexual stimulation to work—you cannot just take the drug and wait for results. Possible side effects include headache, flushing, digestive difficulties, nasal congestion, blurred vision, and light sensitivity. There is also a risk of too-low blood pressure, which can be very dangerous.

Some medications used to treat impotence are administered by self-injection into the base of the penis. These drugs cause blood to be held in the veins in the penis, resulting in erections that last for an hour or more. (Determining the proper dosage is important, as too much can cause painful, long-lasting erections.) Although many men have reported satisfactory results, others find the method to be an unacceptable option.

Vacuum pumps create a vacuum around the penis, causing blood to flow to the area that results in a temporary erection. To maintain the erection, a rubber constriction ring is fitted around the penis, trapping the blood inside. Although the erection is somewhat unsteady, it is sufficient to allow intercourse.

If other treatments are not successful, surgery is an option. Older procedures involve the insertion of a penile implant. Newer surgical procedures treat poor penile blood flow, focusing on the arteries and veins of the penis. The most common of these procedures is the penile artery bypass, which is similar to bypass heart surgery. Keep in mind, however, that the surgeries described here are invasive, and should only be considered if other treatment methods have failed.

## PROBLEMS SPECIFIC TO WOMEN

Compared with the sexual problems associated with diabetes in men, the effects on women are more subtle. This doesn't mean they're any less real, however. The most common sexual problems that women experience are vaginal dryness and yeast infections. Fortunately, while these conditions are uncomfortable, they can be remedied relatively easily.

### *Vaginal Dryness*

The vagina produces a natural lubricant fairly quickly as women become aroused, increasing both lovers' comfort during intercourse. Lubrication also increases the sensitivity of the vaginal lips to touch. Unfortunately, for some women with diabetes, there may not be enough vaginal moistening to make intercourse pleasurable, or even comfortable.

There are a number of factors that contribute to loss of vaginal lubrication in women with diabetes. A primary cause in many women is nerve damage, or neuropathy. Diabetic neuropathy can cause a partial loss of sensation in the genital area, reducing the body's responsiveness to sexual stimulation.

Blood vessel damage—a long-term complication of diabetes—can also cause vaginal lubrication to diminish. When women become aroused, arteries in the genital area open up, increasing blood flow into the area. Some of the fluid portion of the blood passes out of the blood vessels in the vaginal wall and mixes with intercellular fluid, forming a natural lubricant. Circulatory problems resulting from blood vessel damage may decrease blood flow to the vaginal wall, limiting the fluid available for lubrication.

To complicate the situation further, hormonal changes associated with menopause cause persistent vaginal dryness in many women—with or without diabetes—at this stage of life. The sex hormone estrogen promotes normal vaginal lubrication. When estrogen production begins to decline after menopause, the production of vaginal lubricant decreases as well, causing vaginal dryness. Postmenopausal women with diabetes must contend with both the normal age-related loss of lubrication, plus the additional loss often caused by neuropathy or blood vessel damage. And women with poorly controlled diabetes may begin to experience dryness even before the onset of menopause. This is because uncontrolled high blood sugar can lower normal estrogen levels in women, with a resulting loss of vaginal lubrication.

***What to Do About Vaginal Dryness.*** There are a number of commercial lubricants available that can enhance your comfort and pleasure during intercourse. Water-based lubricants, such as K-Y jelly, offer many advantages over other products because they are safe for use in the vagina and wash off easily after sex. Additionally, water-based lubricants are safe for use with latex contraceptives. On the other hand, oil-based lubricants, including those containing petroleum jelly and baby oil, should not be used inside the vagina because they may irritate the vaginal lining. Also, oil-based lubricants have been shown to destroy latex within a very short amount of time, and therefore should *not* be used with latex contraceptives.

Women who are experiencing vaginal dryness due to hormonal changes may want to consider supplemental estrogen in the form of pills, patches, or vaginal creams. If you think estrogen replacement therapy may be the solution to your problem, talk to your doctor. Together you can weigh the benefits against the risks to decide if supplemental estrogen is right for you.

## *Yeast Infections*

*Candida albicans* is a sugar-loving yeast that normally inhabits the mouth, digestive system, genital tract, and skin. A healthy body has the means to keep candida growth under control. As long as the human body has sufficient numbers of "friendly" bacteria, candida remains a benign yeast that neither helps nor harms. If the friendly bacteria are weak and low in numbers, however, candida can develop into a more aggressive, invasive form.

Women with uncontrolled high blood sugar are predisposed to an overgrowth of candida. Why? The presence of an abundance of sugar for the yeast to feed on encourages them to grow. (People whose diets include large quantities of sugar and yeast-based foods also have an increased susceptibility.) Candida infection of the female genital tract causes symptoms such as an odorous vaginal discharge and itching.

***What to Do About Yeast Infections.*** Because candida thrives on sugar in the body, you can decrease the occurrence of infection by practicing tight blood sugar control. Although there are many over-the-counter preparations available to treat yeast infections, you must not treat vaginal infections without reporting them to your doctor. Frequent vaginal yeast infections may be a sign that you're not effectively controlling your blood sugar.

## Psychological Problems

What's your most important sexual organ? Think about this for a while. The correct response is . . . your brain! So if a sexual problem has no physiological cause, then its cause must be psychological. In fact, the psychological variables that affect sexual activity are just as real as the physiological factors. Anxiety, depression, and fear can all form emotional blocks that severely impair sexual enjoyment.

Let's learn about the various psychological problems that may affect sexual relations, and discuss how these obstacles can be overcome.

### POOR SELF-IMAGE

Living with diabetes can certainly affect your self-esteem. Do you feel like a different person now that you have diabetes? Do you like yourself less because of your condition? If your answer to either of these questions is yes, your self-image has suffered as a result of your diabetes. And you may be more fearful of rejection by your partner. As a result, you may reduce sexual activity simply to minimize this chance of rejection.

Why might you perceive yourself as being different as a result of your diabetes? How has diabetes affected your perception of your sexuality? You may feel that you are less masculine or feminine now because of changes in your body. Or perhaps you have gained some weight, either before or since your diagnosis. You may even be afraid to get dressed or undressed in front of your partner.

Dissatisfaction with your appearance can most certainly cause your self-esteem to drop. And you can't truly enjoy sexual intimacy if you don't feel good about yourself. So what's the answer? Consider the changes that have affected you the most, and speak to professionals to learn about things you can do to eliminate or lessen any problems. For example, if you feel bad because you are overweight, work toward becoming more physically fit. (And keep in mind that exercise can really help you manage your diabetes, too!)

Although working on your physical appearance is important to looking good and feeling better, probably the most significant step you can take is to work on your attitude. Tell yourself that nobody's perfect—and nobody expects you to be perfect, either! Feel good about the things that are truly important, and minimize the rest.

## FEAR OF PREGNANCY

Research has shown that withdrawal from sexual activities is sometimes the result of a fear of pregnancy. This can even be a subconscious fear—one that you're not consciously aware of. Whether your reasoning is conscious or unconscious, the avoidance of sex may seem like the best way to avoid getting pregnant.

Why might you be afraid of getting pregnant? There are a number of reasons. You may be concerned that it will affect your condition. You may be concerned that it will be more difficult to control your diabetes, and that your baby will not be born healthy because of this. You may be concerned that you will be less effective as a parent because you have a chronic medical condition. And any or all of these fears can have an impact on your feelings about sex.

If you feel that fear of pregnancy is a problem, speak to your doctor about an appropriate form of birth control. This will help you feel safer, allowing you to relax and enjoy your relationship.

## EMOTIONAL INTERFERENCE

Sexual activity—and sexual desire—may be impaired by a number of emotions. For instance, depression may keep you from having any interest in sex. Anxiety concerning sex itself or the intimacy of your relationship can also hold you back. Certainly, negative emotions don't enhance the pleasure of sexual intimacy!

When negative thoughts and feelings affect sexual desire or performance, it's necessary to get at the root of the cause, and to use coping strategies to eliminate troubling emotions. If anxiety or depression is affecting your sexual well-being, you'll want to improve your attitude. Use some of the thought-changing techniques described earlier in the book. They may be the key to your future happiness!

What else can you do to eliminate psychological obstacles to a fulfilling sex life? A very important part of sexual relationships is communication. If you and your partner can share thoughts and feelings, you'll be in much better shape to work out any problems that may occur as a result of your condition. If necessary, work to alter the ways in which the two of you express your sexual desires. Fully communicate your needs. And remember that problems get worse only when you chronically avoid the issues—not when you openly discuss them and work together to find solutions.

Besides communicating your feelings and fears to your partner, you might also want to discuss any problems with your physician or with other health-care professionals. For instance, perhaps you are concerned about the possibility of hypoglycemia after sexual activity. That thought's probably enough to kill a romantic mood! While hypoglycemia is a potential problem, realize that there are steps you can take to prevent its development—for example, you may need to adjust your medication before sex, or to eat a snack before or after sexual activity.

Everything that's been said in this section assumes that your sexual interest or performance has been affected by psychological problems, and that your partner is suffering as a result. But what if the opposite is true? What if you still have normal sexual desires and normal performance, but your partner is the one who's afraid? Discuss this with your partner. Make sure that you communicate with each other, and be sure to set up ground rules so that you know which sexual activities are okay and which, if any, aren't. And if these one-on-one attempts at working things out don't help, don't hesitate to get some professional assistance. The results will be well worth the effort!

## What If You're Single?

If you are single and dating, your concerns may be different from those of a person who is married or in another type of long-term relationship. For example, you may wonder when the best time is to tell the person you're dating about your condition. Should you mention it right from the start, or not until you're approaching a sexual encounter? In general, most experts believe that you need not say anything from the very beginning. After all, you want to get to know the person first, and you want the person to get to know you. Then, if the relationship seems to be proceeding in the right direction, you may want to consider a comfortable time to mention your condition.

How should you do it? There are as many different ways of saying something as there are people. The one most common piece of advice, though, is to show that you're handling your diabetes. Make it sound as if you're in control. The most frightening thing for a prospective partner is the feeling that you're so overwhelmed by your disease that it's definitely going to have an impact on the relationship.

## And Now, the Climax

When dealing with any sexual problems that result from your diabetes, remember that much can be done to improve both your feelings regarding sex and your enjoyment of the activity. Psychological coping strategies can help you overcome many obstacles to interest and performance. But the most important is open communication with your partner. Even if your sex life becomes less active, you can still have a warm relationship—but not if there are bitter feelings and misgivings. Honest discussions, marked by understanding, are a vital part of coping with sexual problems, just as they are a necessary part of coping with any other aspect of diabetes.

## CHAPTER THIRTY-TWO

# Living with Someone Who Has Diabetes

A chronic medical condition such as diabetes doesn't affect just the person with the disease. It also affects everyone who's close to that person. Those who are in the inner circle are affected most profoundly. They are also in the best position to help the person who is living with diabetes.

Illness can create troubling changes in relationships. If you live with someone who has diabetes, you may now view that person—and even yourself—differently. Maybe you see that person as being more fragile. Perhaps their disorder has reminded you of your own vulnerability. You may feel guilty about their condition, or about your feelings regarding the condition. Maybe you were quite dependent on that person, and now you have to shoulder more responsibility.

What does all this mean? First, you are concerned about the individual with diabetes. You may also feel concerned about the future and possible financial problems. And while you want to do everything you can to support that person, there may be times when it's very difficult for you to contribute. This chapter offers some suggestions to help you take care of your loved one *and* yourself, as you both learn to cope with diabetes.

# How You Can Help the Person with Diabetes

If you are close to someone with diabetes, you have an important job on your hands—a job made up of many components. But what is your job, and how can you best accomplish it? Read on!

## BECOME A LOYAL LEARNER

You can help your friend or loved one simply by learning as much as you can about diabetes and its treatment. This will enable you to provide support and true understanding. Knowing the facts may help you to conquer your fears of the unknown and eliminate your confusion over symptoms, treatments, and side effects.

## ENCOURAGE, DON'T PESTER

There are many ways in which you can help your close friend or family member manage diabetes, without being perceived as a "nag." You can show your support by participating in some aspects of his or her treatment program. For example, you can be an "exercise buddy" and jog, walk, swim, or bike along with your loved one. This will help your friend or relative stick to his or her exercise program. It might just do you some good, too! Also, if your diet consists mainly of nutrient-poor, high-fat foods, you may want to modify *your* eating plan—it can't hurt, right? Try choosing nutritious and delicious meals that your whole family can enjoy together. You may even find some new family favorites! This way, your loved one won't feel "different," or believe that he or she is being deprived of tasty foods.

You may feel frustrated if your loved one does not practice proper self-care. Perhaps he or she is eating poorly, or is not sticking to an approved exercise program, despite your support and encouragement. If this is the case, try to minimize your criticism. Don't be pushy or overprotective; he or she may simply become more resistant to your suggestions. Instead, offer gentle reminders about good self-care skills. Your message is much more likely to get through if it's offered in a kind way.

If the person with diabetes does not stick to the prescribed treatment program, should you tell the physician? That's a hard question to answer. You don't want to overstep your bounds, as this may lead to resentment. At the same time, you don't want to sit back and let your loved one create unnecessary problems.

So what should you do? Play it by ear. Voice your concerns. Explain that you're afraid his or her problems will become worse due to lack of proper treatment. Then listen carefully to his or her response before you contact the physician.

## PROVIDE SUPPORT, NOT PITY

Living with diabetes can be difficult. You may sympathize with your loved one. The sympathy you feel may help you to provide beneficial support. But going overboard with pity can be destructive.

At times your loved one may be too fatigued to do anything. When this happens, do not insist that he or she "get up and do something." That won't help the situation! Instead, try to help out by taking over some of your loved one's responsibilities. This can reduce some of the pressure that he or she may feel to get things done. At the same time, don't relieve your loved one of all responsibilities. In general, if the person is capable of doing something—even if it takes time—let him or her do it. If you feel that he or she is malingering, have an open, honest discussion about this behavior. Your goal is to try to make life as normal as possible for the person with diabetes.

## AVOID OVERPROTECTION

As a family member or close friend, it's very important to be attuned to the needs of your loved one. Don't assume that you must be overprotective or underprotective simply because that's the way you would want others to act if you were ill. Be sure to find out what your loved one needs, and try to act accordingly.

Don't smother the person with diabetes. Sure, you want to help. When your friend or loved one is tired, for instance, you can help out by taking over some of his or her chores. Make sure to give the person enough space to regain control over his or her life. How? When your loved one is no longer tired, be sure to let him or her return to a normal routine. Don't insist that the person rest! Have faith in your special someone. That person will rest when he or she really doesn't feel well.

What about accompanying your loved one on doctors' visits? If he or she asks, you may want to go along for the ride. As discussed in chapter 29, it's an excellent idea to have four ears, rather than two, listening when the doctor explains about the diabetes itself or details treatment options. However, if the person wants to go alone, don't try to tag along.

What's the bottom line here? You should work with your loved one to set ground rules. Talk about your interest in being as supportive as you possibly can, and ask what you can do to help. Things will move more smoothly once you know what to do and when to do it. Even if no clear-cut answers emerge, at least you'll have shared some constructive communication. This will help you handle future problems. Just remember that your loved one has the final say in all decisions.

## KEEP TALKING

What's the best way to talk to your loved one? Unfortunately, because everybody's different and because needs change along with moods and circumstances, there's no way to know for sure. At certain times, you may feel that it's best to respond with sympathy and understanding. At other times, it may be best to ignore the situation and walk away. You'll have to play things by ear, remaining attuned to your partner's needs as much as possible.

However you decide to talk to your special someone, by all means, *keep talking*! The key to maintaining harmony is communication. Why is this so valuable? Because communication will help you learn how your loved one feels, both physically and emotionally. And you'll be better able to help when you know how he or she feels. This doesn't mean that the conversations will always be pleasant. Talking about diabetes management, depression, or fear isn't very enjoyable, especially if you don't have any solutions. However, any difficulties will be overshadowed by the feeling of closeness that results from shared experiences and concerns.

As much as you would like to talk to your loved one, there may be times when he or she will not be willing to respond. When this happens, it's fine to reassure the person that you're aware of this. You'll be there to listen when he or she needs a sympathetic ear.

### TAKE CARE OF YOURSELF, TOO!

Although you've learned a great deal about coping with diabetes from reading this book, so far little attention has been paid to the problems that diabetes poses for friends and family members of the person who is ill. You may experience many of the same emotions and changes in lifestyle experienced by your loved one, but feel more helpless because everything is happening *around* you rather than *to* you. You may experience depression, anxiety, or anger. Or you may feel guilty if you have trouble adjusting to new chores and responsibilities, or a new daily routine.

How can you cope with these feelings? Accept that it's okay to experience these feelings, but don't allow them to linger. Restructure your thinking. Remind yourself that you are doing what you can to help your loved one. Don't forget that you also need—and deserve—nurturing attention. Don't be afraid to reach out and get it. You can benefit from the same kinds of support groups as your loved one. Don't hesitate to take advantage of them.

## A Supportive Synopsis

True, diabetes is not affecting your body. But it is certainly affecting you in other ways. There will be times when your loved one needs a helping hand, a sympathetic ear, or a shoulder to cry on. Naturally, you want to do all of this and more for your special someone. But you can't be strong for others if you don't take care of yourself, as well. So remember to take some time out for *you.* When you're refreshed, you'll be all the more ready to help your loved one cope with diabetes.

## CHAPTER THIRTY-THREE

# Children with Diabetes

How did you react when your child was diagnosed with diabetes? Did you feel angry? Did you feel numb? Did you break down and cry?

It's common for parents to have trouble coping with a child's illness. Raising a healthy child is challenging enough, after all! As a parent, you are responsible for your child's physical and emotional well-being. So a diagnosis of diabetes can be devastating for your family. You may fear that you'll never be able to deal with the medical reality of the condition. You may wonder if your family can possibly adapt to the lifestyle changes a disease such as diabetes requires. And, like so many parents of children with diabetes, you may worry that your child will never lead a "normal" life.

How can you begin to help your child cope with diabetes? Accept the fact that diabetes won't just "go away," but remember that diabetes management must not take over your family's life. Love, guide, and discipline your child as if diabetes were not a factor. And tell yourself that a diagnosis of diabetes is not totally negative—people grow and change not only when things are going well, but also during times of adversity.

This chapter will first look at what you can do to help yourself cope with the problems involved in caring for a child with diabetes. Remember, there will be times when you'll have to reach out and get help for yourself so that you can be as strong as you possibly can for your family. Then, we'll look at how you can give your child the tools and self-confidence it takes to manage his or her own care.

## Coping with Your Emotions

When your child was first diagnosed with diabetes, you may not have been able to react at all; you may have felt "separated" from your emotions. Or you may have felt intense anger, sadness, fear, guilt, or despair. Maybe you even felt relieved to find out the cause of your child's illness. Chances are, you experienced each of these emotions at some point after the initial diagnosis.

Of all the feelings you might have experienced after the diagnosis, guilt and fear are probably the most destructive emotions. Why? These two emotions can interfere with your acceptance of diabetes and its treatment as a part of your life. And your ability to care for your child ultimately depends on your acceptance of his or her condition. So let's take a moment to discuss guilt and fear, and the steps you can take to overcome these emotions.

### GUILT

Because type 1 diabetes—the most common type of diabetes diagnosed in children—can be hereditary, many parents are afraid that they did something to contribute to their child's illness. Additionally, some parents believe that if they had taken better care of their child, the condition would never have developed. These are the kinds of negative thoughts that contribute to feelings of guilt.

Your feelings of guilt will not positively affect your ability to care for your child. Rather, guilt can lower your self-image and exhaust your emotional resources, leaving you with less of the emotional energy you need to help your child cope. So if you catch yourself feeling guilty because your child has diabetes, work on restructuring your thinking. Instead of telling yourself that you're a "bad" parent because your child developed diabetes, remind yourself of how much you love your child. Ask yourself if you've ever done anything that a "good" parent might do. (You're sure to come up with more than one example!)

In learning to overcome your feelings of guilt, it's important not to dwell on what might have been had your child not developed diabetes. Instead, focus on the present and the future. Concentrate on learning how to help your child cope with diabetes. The idea is to turn your mind's negative thoughts into reasonable, positive ones.

As you learn to cope with diabetes in your family, never underestimate the benefits that support groups have to offer. Groups provide a forum for the exchange of feelings and ideas. You'll hear how others are dealing with feelings of guilt, and gain valuable information and strategies to help you conquer this destructive emotion. Most important, support groups remind you that you're not alone—and it's much easier to live with a difficult problem when you know that you're not alone.

## FEAR

When you first learned about your child's condition, were you overwhelmed by feelings of fear? It's certainly natural to feel afraid when someone you love is diagnosed with a serious illness. And when that illness requires so much care and so many lifestyle changes—as diabetes does—you may be fearful that you won't be able to provide the kind of care your child needs to grow up healthy and well-adjusted. "How will I ever be able to give him insulin injections?" "Can I really learn to check her blood glucose?" "I'll never get him to eat the right foods!" "How can I teach her to take care of herself?" "What will school be like for him?" "What if her condition gets worse?"

Education is the key to overcoming your fears about your child's well-being. Learn as much as you can about diabetes—what it is, how it affects your child, and how it's treated. Knowing the facts will help you feel more confident in your approach to treatment, and will enable you to communicate more effectively with your child's health-care team. Perhaps most important, you'll be well-equipped to teach your child about the importance of good diabetes management.

When you first set out to gather information on diabetes, keep in mind that you don't need to learn everything all at once—otherwise you can easily become overwhelmed. Some parents get so caught up in learning about diabetes that the disease seems to take over their lives! Don't allow this to happen. Your goal is to adapt to diabetes as a normal part of your life, not to make diabetes treatment the focus of your life.

## Your Child's Treatment Program

Until your child is old enough to handle diabetes management, you're going to be responsible for every aspect of his or her treatment program. This means that you will have to talk to the health-care team, administer insulin injections, monitor blood glucose, count carbohydrates, and encourage your child to exercise. You will have to be on the alert for warning signs of hypoglycemia, and be prepared to treat the complication. And you'll have to know when symptoms of illness are serious enough to contact your child's treatment team.

If all of this seems a little daunting, take comfort in the fact that diabetes management will get easier as it becomes more routine. Remember that you can rely on your child's treatment team—they are there to show you the ropes and answer your questions, and they're just a phone call away. Ideally, you will also have the full support of your family and close friends. Relatives and friends can provide essential emotional support, and can help out with chores and other responsibilities if you start to feel overwhelmed.

Now let's take a look at some of the ways you can ensure the success of your child's diabetes treatment program.

### ESTABLISH A GOOD DOCTOR-PATIENT-PARENT RELATIONSHIP

Your child's primary-care physician is the hub of the wheel as far as diabetes treatment is concerned. He or she takes responsibility for your child's overall health, determines your child's target blood glucose level, coordinates the efforts of the treatment team, and provides guidelines for any lifestyle changes that may be beneficial or necessary.

Of course you want the very best for your child, so you must choose a doctor in whom you have confidence medically. This is only part of the equation, however. Just as important, you'll want to find someone with whom you and your child are comfortable personally. Naturally, you should feel confident that the doctor can address your questions and concerns. But you should also be assured that the physician you choose has the consideration and patience to address your child's concerns. Make sure that your child feels comfortable asking questions. This will encourage your child to become an effective self-advocate as he or she takes over responsibility for diabetes management.

## GET SCHOOL PERSONNEL INVOLVED

Obviously, you can't be with your child every minute of every day. When school starts, you'll have to entrust your child's care to teachers and other school personnel. Open communication with school personnel will help ensure that your child has a comfortable, safe, and happy school experience.

Before you send your son or daughter off to school, contact the child's teacher. If the teacher is not knowledgeable about diabetes and its treatment, it will be helpful to provide some background information about the disease. Also, explain that most children with diabetes do best if they eat several meals at the same time each day, so your child might need a midmorning or midafternoon snack.

It's a good idea to prepare a written plan that includes:

- When your child's blood sugar should be tested.
- Warning signs of hypoglycemia.
- Instructions for treating hypoglycemia.
- How to notify you in case of a medical emergency.
- How to contact your child's physician in case of a medical emergency.
- Your child's preferred snacks and "safe" party foods.

Unless you child's management plan requires an insulin injection prior to lunch, insulin is usually not administered at school. The school nurse will take responsibility for giving your child insulin shots (if necessary), and monitoring blood glucose at the appropriate times.

When you talk with your child's teacher, emphasize the idea that your child should not receive special treatment. Most school children just want to feel "normal"—they don't want their peers to see them as being different. Your child will be expected to complete his or her own work, and should be rewarded or disciplined like his or her classmates—as if diabetes were not a factor. The teacher should not allow your child to get away with behavior for which other students would be disciplined. Not only would this do a disservice to your child, but it might foster peer conflicts.

## ENCOURAGE COMMUNICATION

As you help your child learn to cope with diabetes, it's essential to keep the lines of communication open. Why is this so important? Only through communication will you learn how your son or daughter feels, physically and emotionally. And only by knowing how he or she feels will you be able to help.

How can you encourage communication? Try setting aside some special time when you can chat with your child. Make it a routine—a standing date for good conversation. And you don't just have to talk about diabetes. Take an interest in what's going on in your child's life apart from diabetes. But let your child know that you'll be ready to talk about diabetes and treatment issues when he or she feels comfortable discussing these topics.

What if your child is reluctant to talk? Don't try to force your child to open up if he or she isn't ready. Reassure your son or daughter that you'll be available to listen when you're called upon. If you remind your child of this often enough, you can be sure that he or she will come to you when the time is right.

As your child grows older—particularly as he or she enters into the teenage years—communication may become a bit more strained. Remember, this can happen in any parent–child relationship, whether or not the adolescent has diabetes. We'll discuss the special problems that parents and adolescents face later on in this chapter.

## AVOID PARENTAL PITFALLS

Let's take a moment to consider some of the goals of diabetes management. Obviously, you are concerned about your child's physical well-being. Until your son or daughter is old enough to assume responsibility for self-care, you will be in charge of keeping his or her blood sugar within a target range. But remember that you are responsible for your child's emotional well-being, as well. In the long term, you want to know that your child will have the self-control and self-confidence necessary for a normal life.

Above all else, you must make sure your child feels normal and accepted. Emphasize the child rather than the illness. Don't refer to your son or daughter as "diabetic." Instead, think of him or her as a normal child who just happens to have diabetes. This way, your child will grow up with an identity that is separate from the illness.

As with everything in life, balance is key. You want to teach your child the importance of good self-care skills, but stress the fact that diabetes management should not be all-consuming. And you need to be ready to relinquish control as your child begins to demonstrate the maturity to take over his or her own care.

Does this seem like a tall order? It doesn't have to be, as long as you avoid the following pitfalls:

- **Overindulgence.** Some parents believe that the rigors of self-care are too intense for their child to handle, so they offer special treats while providing little discipline. As a result, the child learns poor self-care skills, and may feel incapable of handling self-care when the time comes.

- **Overprotection.** In this case, the parents are so worried about their child's health that they continue to handle most of the details of diabetes management, even when their child is old enough to assume responsibility for treatment. A child raised in this type of environment tends to be overdependent, lacking the self-confidence necessary to be fully responsible for self-care.

- **Indifference.** Indifferent parents are the opposite extreme—they don't fuss *enough* over their child's care, and don't provide the discipline and support necessary for the child to learn good self-care skills. The danger here is that the child may "rebel" and seek attention through negative behaviors, such as skipping insulin injections, "forgetting" to do blood glucose tests, or eating the wrong foods. Obviously, these behaviors can have some very harmful physical effects.

No, you're not perfect. (Who is?) You won't always make the "right" decisions when it comes to parenting. Even parents of healthy children struggle with issues such as discipline versus indulgence and overprotection versus indifference. Just don't lose sight of the bigger picture. Overall, your goal is to raise your child to be a responsible, well-adjusted adult. And when all's said and done, isn't that what every parent wants?

## EXPLORE PROFESSIONAL COUNSELING

Making the adjustment to living with diabetes can be very difficult for a child, especially if any restrictions imposed by the condition interfere with normal activities. Some children may react by denying that the condition exists. They may believe that if they ignore diabetes, it will just go away. So they may continue to eat the wrong foods, or refuse or "forget" to take their medication. Clearly, this is harmful behavior. Other children may become angry and lash out—temper tantrums are not uncommon among children who are learning to live with diabetes. Depression may also be more likely to occur in children with diabetes. Naturally, you want to do everything you can to help your child. But sometimes, even a parent's support and understanding are not enough.

If your child is having a great deal of difficulty coping with diabetes—if learning to live with the disease is just too painful—then professional counseling may help. You child may feel that he or she can be totally honest with a counselor, and can express feelings that may otherwise remain hidden. At the same time, the child can get feedback that can help him or her better deal with these feelings. If you don't know an appropriate professional, you can get a referral from your child's physician, from your local chapter of the American Diabetes Association, or from a local hospital or professional organization.

A support group can also help your child overcome negative feelings about diabetes. There your child will meet kids his or her own age who are learning to cope with the same challenges and issues. Support groups can provide a great feeling of fellowship and inspiration. Your child can share his or her feelings more openly in this kind of nurturing, supportive environment. Check out the list of resource groups on page 347 to locate an appropriate resource group for your child. You may also want to contact sources such as local hospitals, schools of psychology or social work, or religious organizations.

## CONSIDER DIABETES CAMPS

Summer camps for children with diabetes can be an excellent way to educate children about diabetes and self-care, and provide a positive, upbeat environment in which children can socialize with others with diabetes. These camps provide fun, recreation, and learning as well as good consistent treatment for diabetes and further information about diabetes and its control for the campers. A list of camps that cater to children with diabetes can be obtained from the American Diabetes Association. You can also get valuable information online at the Children with Diabetes Web site: www.childrenwithdiabetes.com.

## Transferring Control

The age at which children are ready to take over self-care responsibilities varies from child to child. Generally, experts agree that children can assume many of the responsibilities of diabetes management at around the age of twelve. However, children can become involved in diabetes care at a much earlier age. For instance, even very young children can have a say in treatment matters. You can encourage participation by allowing your child to pick an injection site, read the blood glucose monitor, and choose healthy foods for meals.

Make diabetes management a regular part of your daily routine. Set a good example—teach you child that compliance and consistency are essential to diabetes management, and emphasize the idea that the reward of his or her hard work is good health. This way, when your child is ready to take on the challenge of self-care, he or she will already possess some good habits.

It's best to ease your child into accepting full responsibility for self-care. Allow your son or daughter to take over more tasks as he or she demonstrates greater intellectual and emotional maturity. But continue to oversee your child's treatment program. Be vigilant and remind your son or daughter if he or she neglects any aspect of self-care. Emphasize the idea that this is a constructive team effort so that your child will not resent your involvement. As he or she accepts more of the responsibility, accept the fact that your primary role is to provide encouragement and support.

## Handling Sibling Rivalry

Sibling rivalry is normal in any family, whether or not one child has a chronic illness. So when diabetes comes into play, it's easy to see how rivalry among brothers and sisters can develop.

When one of your children has a serious illness such as diabetes, the other children in your family will definitely be affected. They may resent the extra attention that they feel is being lavished on the child with diabetes, and begin to believe that their needs are secondary. This problem is certainly compounded if friends and relatives fuss over the one child. Brothers and sisters may think that the whole illness is being blown out of proportion—that the child with diabetes is making a big deal out of nothing, just to get some attention.

How can you keep sibling rivalry from breeding bad feelings among your children? Good communication is definitely key. Let your children know that you understand why they might feel left out, and that you certainly do not intend to push them aside. Remind them that they're every bit as important as the child with diabetes, and that you love all of your children equally. And make sure they know that you'll be available to listen if they feel their needs aren't being met.

## Dealing with Adolescents

Adolescence is just not easy. It's a time of insecurity, sensitivity, rapid physical and emotional growth, and friendships made and broken. It's a time when the teenager struggles to forge a new identity, while attempting to fit in with his or her peers. And, as so many parents know, it can be a time of rebellion, as the child begins to crave more independence.

For an adolescent with diabetes, these trying times can be even more difficult. Let's learn a little bit about the trials and tribulations of adolescence, and how diabetes can compound these problems.

### THE NEED FOR ACCEPTANCE

As discussed earlier, children with diabetes don't want to be different—they want to be a part of the crowd. Peer acceptance becomes even more important in the adolescent years. Remember, social relationships are very important at this stage of life—friendships eclipse all the other facets of daily life. So a teenager with diabetes may try very hard to hide his or her condition from classmates and friends. Or the teenager may be more reluctant to develop social relationships because of concerns about feeling different.

If you sense that your child is feeling lonely or excluded, talk about it. Remind your teen that *everyone* is different. It's our differences that make us unique individuals. Ask your child to think of some other teens who have to deal with their own differences. Your teen will come to realize that his or her schoolmates aren't as similar as they appear, even though they may look and act alike.

Your child may have a hard time deciding whether or not to tell friends about diabetes. He or she may be concerned that this information will hurt friendships, that friends may be afraid or upset—even hostile—when they hear the news. Some friends may even be scared that they'll "catch" diabetes. So how can you help your son or daughter in this situation? Remind your child that he or she may feel more relaxed if one or two close friends knew about the problem. Your child may feel pressured to hide the truth from friends, and this can certainly take its toll on his or her emotional well-being. Reassure you child that true friends will take the announcement in stride, and won't let diabetes stand in the way of a good friendship.

Perhaps your teen wants to let friends know about the situation, but can't find the right words. If this is the case, then you'll need to do some brainstorming. Sit down with your son or daughter and think of ways to talk about diabetes. Once your teen has settled on a comfortable way to approach the topic, spend some time rehearsing what he or she will say. If your child is uncomfortable participating in this kind of discussion with you, you might want to ask your child's health-care team for assistance. Members of the health-care team may have some experience helping children with diabetes educate others about the disease.

In some cases, your child's diabetes may, in fact, be the cause of broken friendships. Because of some of the restrictions imposed by diabetes and diabetes management, your child might not be able to spend as much time with friends as desired. He or she might not be able to go out as often as friends do. Your child's friends may become annoyed or irritated by these restrictions, and may decide not to bother to maintain the friendship.

If your child loses a friend because of factors related to diabetes, ask your child why he or she thinks this happened. For example, did your child inadvertently push the friend away? Could the friendship have been saved if the friend knew a little more about diabetes? Or was the friend simply uninterested in learning about the condition? It's important to examine these possibilities, so that your child can learn from the situation (although it's certainly a painful lesson).

## THE NEED FOR INDEPENDENCE

Adolescents want to be more independent. They are approaching adulthood, and feel that they should be treated as adults, with all of the freedoms that come with the territory. Naturally, it's difficult for parents to begin to let go as their children grow older. When teenagers demand more freedoms than their parents are ready or willing to concede, the result is rarely a healthy compromise. Instead, the parents usually find themselves with a rebellious teen on their hands.

Rebellion is a part of growing up. It's the result of a child's attempts to define a new identity as an adult. Again, this stage of adolescence may be more painful and volatile for children with diabetes. Why? Because the natural tendency of any parent is to become overprotective when a child is sick. A teen with diabetes may resent what he or she perceives as interference on the part of the parents. This is made worse by the fact that rapid physical changes during adolescence cause blood sugar levels to fluctuate more frequently, resulting in the need for close monitoring and perhaps more supervision. Clearly, closer supervision is the *last* thing a teenager wants at a time when independence is of utmost importance!

How can you resolve these conflicts? Realize that your teenager expects support and understanding during these trying times. Let your child be responsible for self-care. Try to keep an eye on his or her progress, but don't send the message that you don't trust your child. Even when your child pushes too hard, try not to interfere. Some way or another, your child must learn what he or she can or cannot do. If your child is forgetful or careless in the approach to self-care, engage him or her in constructive discussions. You'll find that gentle reminders are much more effective than put-downs or confrontations.

Some parents try to protect their adolescents by withholding information about their diabetes. This is not a good idea. If you expect your child to be responsible for diabetes management, then he or she needs to know all the facts—even if the truth is a little scary. By attempting to protect your child, you will actually be hindering his or her adjustment to living with diabetes. This can breed anger and bitterness, which can have serious long-term effects on your relationship.

Rebellion may occasionally lead to more serious physical problems for your adolescent. Why? Because a rebellious teenager may be less diligent with diabetes self-care. On occasion, the adolescent may even deliberately try to make the condition worse, by eating the wrong foods or by taking insulin incorrectly or inconsistently.

There are many reasons why your teen might engage in these negative behaviors. Some teens neglect their health when they want more attention. Others might do it just for spite. Still others neglect to follow their care programs as a way of avoiding the situation altogether. Before you can deal with this behavior, you need to understand your child's motives for acting out. Then you can take steps to improve communication. Try to make your child understand that these negative behaviors are extremely dangerous, and that there are healthier ways to express feelings. If you are unable to reach your child, try talking to your child's health-care team. Members of the health-care team will have more experience in dealing with rebellious teens, and they can offer invaluable advice.

## QUESTIONS ABOUT THE FUTURE

As your child gets older, he or she may become troubled by questions about the future. You child might ask "Will I be able to finish my education?" "Will I be able to get married?" "Will I be able to have children?" "Will I be able to lead a normal life?"

How can you help your child feel confident about the future? Remind your child that good self-care now will lead to good health in the future. Emphasize the fact that millions of people are living rich, full lives despite diabetes, and there's no reason why your child can't also. It might be helpful to do a little research—together, you and your child can learn about famous actors, politicians, and other high-profile figures who are coping successfully with diabetes.

# In Conclusion

Because your child has diabetes, you will have to deal with special challenges that parents of healthy children will never face. Initially, you'll have to take full responsibility for every aspect of your child's treatment program. But as your child grows older, you must relinquish some of this control—and that may not be easy.

So how can you learn to let go? One of the most important things you can do is to get your child involved in treatment early on. Set a good example for consistency in self-care to help your son or daughter develop good habits. And remind your child that excellent self-care skills are rewarded with continued good health. When your child is mature enough to begin taking some responsibilities of diabetes management, transfer control gradually, so that he or she will not feel overwhelmed. Each small success will help give your child the confidence necessary to assume total responsibility for self-care.

# On to the Future

Well, you've just about finished this book. We've covered a lot of information about diabetes. Ongoing research continues to test new medical techniques that may be able to treat the condition, as well as further improve the quality of life for people with diabetes.

There's a lot of exciting research in diabetes going on all over the world. The changes that have taken place in diabetes treatment over the past ten to twenty years have been phenomenal. And future changes promise to be even more exciting. Perhaps by the time you read this, some drug or treatment may have proven itself to be more successful than ones discussed within these pages. It remains to be seen which new developments may improve your life with diabetes. But it's nice to know that people continue to work on the problem.

Although it would be impossible to discuss every conceivable problem related to diabetes, I hope that what you've read will help you develop your own strategies for coping. Because things change, and something that troubles you one day may not trouble you the next (and vice versa), this book should be used as a resource. Whenever you have questions about how to cope with a certain aspect of diabetes, consult these pages. If you have any comments, information you feel is important, or additional questions, feel free to write to me in care of the publisher.

Until such time as there no longer is a medical condition called diabetes, keep coping the best you can. Remember that despite diabetes, you can *always* improve the quality of your life. So for now, look brightly ahead, act proudly, and enjoy life as best you can. I wish all of my readers the very best of health and happiness!

# For Further Reading

The following books—which provide more information on the material presented in this book, and focus on other topics, as well—may help you cope with the various aspects of living with diabetes. By no means should you limit yourself to the books listed below. Many other publications also examine diabetes treatment, the challenges of living with a chronic illness, and other subjects that may be of interest to you. Don't hesitate to take advantage of all the information available to you at your local library or bookstore.

Beaser, R. *The Joslin Guide to Diabetes*. New York: Simon & Shuster, 1995.

Beatty, M. *My Sister Rose Has Diabetes*. Santa Fe, N.M.: Health Press, 1997.

Betschart, J. *In Control: A Guide for Teens with Diabetes*. Minneapolis: Chronimed Publishing, 1995.

Betschart, J. *It's Time to Learn About Diabetes*. Minneapolis: Chronimed Publishing, 1995.

Brackenridge, B., and R. Rubin. *Sweet Kids: How to Balance Diabetes Control and Good Nutrition with Family Peace*. ADA, 1996.

Breslin, D. *Free Yourself From Pain*. New York: Simon & Schuster, 1986.

Cavaiani, Mabel. *The New Diabetic Cookbook, Second Edition.* Chicago: Contemporary Books, 1994.

Franz, M. *Exchanges for All Occasions, Third Edition.* Minneapolis: Chronimed Publishing, 1993.

Hess, M., and K. Middleton. *The Art of Cooking for the Diabetic.* New York: Signet, 1998.

Juliano, J., and D. Young. *The Diabetic's Innovative Cookbook.* New York: Henry Holt & Company, 1994.

Krumholz, H., and R. Phillips. *No Ifs, Ands, or Butts.* New York: Avery Publishing Group, 1993.

Lazarus, A. *In the Mind's Eye.* New York: Rawson Associates, 1977.

Linchitz, R. *Life Without Pain.* New York: Addison-Wesley, 1987.

Malder, L. *Sarah and Paffle: A Story for Children About Diabetes.* New York: Magination Press, 1992.

McAuliffe, A. *Growing Up with Diabetes: What Children Want Their Parents to Know.* Minneapolis: Chronimed Publishing, 1998.

McDaniel, L. *All the Days of Her Life.* New York: Bantam Books, 1994.

Miller, J. *Grilled Cheese at Four O'Clock in the Morning.* ADA, 1988.

Nathan, D. *Diabetes.* New York: Times Books, 1997.

Nemanic, A., G. Kauth, and M. Franz. *Diabetes Care Made Easy.* IDC Publishing, 1992.

Phillips, R. *Control Your Pain!: 169 Painless Strategies for Taking Charge of Your Body.* New York: Balance, 1996.

Saudek, C., R. Rubin, and C. Shump. *The Johns Hopkins Guide to Diabetes.* Baltimore: The Johns Hopkins University Press, 1997.

Simineriol, L., and J. Betschart. *Raising a Child with Diabetes.* ADA, 1995.

# Resource Groups

The following groups can provide you with more information on diabetes, suggest helpful books and videos, direct you to support groups, and inform you of other valuable services. Feel free to contact these organizations and benefit from their expertise.

American Association of Diabetes Educators
100 West Monroe Street
Fourth Floor
Chicago, IL 60603-1901
(312) 424-2426
www.aadenet.org

American Chronic Pain Association
P.O. Box 850
Rocklin, CA 95677
(916) 632-0922

American Diabetes Association
1660 Duke Street
Alexandria, VA 22314-0592
(800) 342-2383 or (703) 549-1500
http://www.diabetes.org

American Dietetic Association
216 West Jackson Boulevard
Chicago, IL 60606-6995
(800) 366-1655
http://www.eatright.org

Children with Diabetes on-line community
http://www.childrenwithdiabetes.com

Juvenile Diabetes Foundation
120 Wall Street
19th Floor
New York, NY 10005
(800) JDF-CURE

National Chronic Pain Outreach Association
7979 Old Georgetown Road, Suite 100
Bethesda, MD 20814
(301) 652-4948
or
P.O. Box 274
Millboro, VA 24460
(540) 997-5004

Triumph Over Pain Foundation
1341 West Folterton Parkway
Suite 120
Chicago, IL 60614
(773) 327-5198

# Index